CURRENT PEDIATRIC DRUGS

Fredric D. Burg, MD

Vice Dean of Education
University of Pennsylvania School of Medicine
Professor of Pediatrics
Children's Hospital of Philadelphia
Philadelphia, Pennsylvania

Jeffrey A. Bourret, MS, RPh

Director of Pharmacy
University of Pennsylvania Medical Center
Hospital of the University of Pennsylvania
Clinical Assistant Professor
Philadelphia College of Pharmacy and Science
Philadelphia, Pennsylvania

W.B. SAUNDERS COMPANY
A Division of Harcourt Brace & Company
Philadelphia London Toronto Montreal Sydney Tokyo

W.B. SAUNDERS COMPANY

A Division of Harcourt Brace & Company

The Curtis Center
Independence Square West
Philadelphia, Pa. 19106

Library of Congress Cataloging-in-Publication Data

Burg, Fredric D. (Fredric David),
Current pediatric drugs / Fredric D. Burg, Jeffrey A. Bourret.
p. cm.
ISBN 0–7216–4574–7
1. Pediatric pharmacology—Handbooks, manuals. etc.
I. Bourret, Jeffrey A. II. Title.
[DNLM: 1. Drug Therapy—in infancy & childhood—handbooks. WS 39 B954c 1993]
RJ560.B87 1994
615.5′8′083—dc20 93-28372

International Edition 0-7216-4807-X

CURRENT PEDIATRIC DRUGS ISBN 0–7216–4574–7

Printed in the United States of America

Last digit is the print number: 9 8 7 6 5 4 3 2 1

Dosage Notice

Every effort has been made by the author to check generic and trade names and to verify drug doses as correct according to the standards accepted at the time of publication. The ultimate responsibility lies with the prescribing physician, on the basis of his or her professional experience and knowledge of the patient to determine dosages and the best course of treatment for the patient. The reader is advised to check the product information currently provided by the manufacturer of each drug to be administered to ascertain any changes in drug dosage, method of administration or contraindications. In no case can the institution with which the author is affiliated or the publisher be held responsible for the views expressed in this book. Please call any errors to the attention of the author.

Contents

Preface

This handbook is a companion reference to the fourteenth edition of *Current Pediatric Therapy.* In it clinically significant drug information is made readily accessible to prescribers in their work environments. Data on the medications most commonly prescribed in the treatment of pediatric illness are presented concisely for quick retrieval.

The clinical tables in the second part of the book were taken from *Current Pediatric Therapy* and are arranged alphabetically by diagnosis for easy reference.

Because this book is a new feature of *Current Pediatric Therapy,* either of the authors would greatly appreciate suggestions on how this formulary can be improved to meet your practice needs.

Fredric D. Burg
Jeffrey A. Bourret

Medication Error Prevention Guidelines

1. Stay abreast of new developments in medication through the literature, consulting with pharmacists and other physicians, and continuing medical education.
2. Review existing drug therapy for each patient before prescribing new medication to ascertain possible drug interactions.
3. Be familiar with the medication-ordering system of your hospital or practice setting, including its procedure for new-drug orders and its medication administration schedule.
4. Make sure each drug order is complete and accurate and includes the desired therapeutic outcome.
5. Strive for clarity: reduce ambiguity by avoiding abbreviations; specify exact dosages; use standard nomenclature; avoid decimals, or precede them with a zero for quantities less than one; and *never* use a zero after a terminal decimal (write 5 ml, not 5.0 ml).
6. Print or type orders if you cannot write legibly.
7. Avoid oral drug orders. If you must use them, dictate slowly and clearly.
8. Prescribe drugs for oral administration whenever possible.
9. Explain medication to the patient, including any special precautions and possible allergic or hypersensitivity reactions.
10. Periodically evaluate the need for each patient's continued drug therapy.
11. Make sure instructions for "hold" orders are clear.

Format for Drug Listing

The following format has been used to organize the information provided for the prescriber for each drug product described:

Tetracycline

SYNONYM: Achromycin, Panmycin, Sumycin

CLASS: Tetracycline

DOSAGE FORM:
Capsules: 250 mg, 500 mg
Injection: for IM use only: 100 mg, 250 mg
Injection: for IV use only: 500 mg
Suspension: Oral, 125 mg/5 ml

SELECTED DOSAGES:
Children >8 Years of Age: Usual oral dosage: 25–50 mg/kg daily given in 2–4 divided doses. Alternatively, some clinicians recommend that children receive 0.6–1.2 g/m^2 daily. The usual IV dosage is 12 mg/kg daily, given in 2 divided doses, but 10–20 mg/kg may be given daily depending on the severity of the infection. The usual IM dosage is 15–25 mg/kg daily, given in 2 or 3 divided doses with a maximum dosage of 250 mg as a single daily injection.

COMMON SIDE EFFECTS: Dose-related GI effects, including nausea, vomiting, diarrhea, bulky loose stools, anorexia, flatulence, abdominal discomfort, epigastric burning and distress, photosensitivity.

SELECTED DRUG INTERACTIONS: Cations (antacids containing aluminum, calcium, or magnesium), drugs affecting GI pH, oral anticoagulants, kaolin, pectin, barbiturates, phenytoin, carbamazepine, lithium.

CAUTIONS: Tetracyclines should not be used in women during pregnancy or in children <9 years of age unless other appropriate drugs are ineffective or are contraindicated. The American Academy of Pediatrics recommends that tetracyclines be used only in children who are ≥9 years of age, except under unusual circumstances. Their use could result in retardation of skeletal development and bone growth in the fetus or child, or in hypoplasia and permanent yellow-gray to brown discoloration of the teeth if used during pregnancy or in children ≤4–6 months of age.

- **Generic drug names** are used to list drugs alphabetically. In addition, common brand names of drugs are cross-referenced throughout the handbook.
- **Synonyms** represent trade or brand names, common names, or abbreviations by which the drug is also identified.
- **Class** describes the classification(s) the drug has been assigned to. Additional information can be obtained by referring to specific chapters in the forteenth edition of *Current Pediatric Therapy.*
- **Dosage Form** refers to available dosage forms, concentration, and dosage form size (e.g., 2 mg/ml, 1 ml vial refers to a 1 ml vial with concentration of 2 mg/ml)
- **Selected Dosages** include some but not all recommendations for drug dosages. Attempts have been made to include dosages for the most frequently treated conditions. Readers should refer to the comparative dosing tables in the second part of this guide for information on dosages for additional conditions for which a drug is used by clinicians in the field.
- **Common Side Effects** include those side effects most commonly reported or believed to be clinically significant.
- **Selected Drug Interactions** include those interactions thought to be clinically significant.
- **Cautions** include statements related to a particular drug that should be considered when prescribing an agent to reduce the potential for adverse experiences with the use of the drug.
- **Controlled Substance** the Drug Enforcement Agency controlled drug schedule (C-II through C-V) is indicated.

Alphabetical Drug Listing

Acetaminophen
Acetazolamide
Acetohydroxamic Acid
Acetylcysteine
Acyclovir
Albuterol
Amantadine Hydrochloride
Amikacin
Amiloride Hydrochloride
Aminophylline
Amitriptyline Hydrochloride
Amoxicillin
Amoxicillin Clavulanic Acid
Ampicillin
Amrinone Lactate
Aspirin
Atenolol
Azathioprine
Captopril
Carbamazepine
Cefaclor
Cefixime
Cefotaxime
Ceftazidime
Ceftriaxone
Cephalexin
Cephalothin
Chlorothiazide
Ciprofloxacin
Clomipramine
Clonidine Hydrochloride
Codeine Phosphate
Cyclophosphamide
Desipramine Hydrochloride
Dextroamphetamine Sulfate
Diazepam
Diazoxide
Dicyclomine Hydrochloride
Digoxin
Diphenhydramine Hydrochloride
Dobutamine Hydrochloride
Dopamine Hydrochloride
Doxycycline
Enalapril
Ferrous Sulfate
Epinephrine
Furosemide
Gentamicin Sulfate
Globulin, Immune Serum, Intravenous
Haloperidol
Heparin Sodium
Hepatitis B Vaccine
Hydralazine Hydrochloride
Hydrochlorothiazide
Hydromorphone
Hydroxyzine
Ibuprofen
Imipramine Hydrochloride
Isoproterenol Hydrochloride
Labetalol Hydrochloride
Lidocaine
Lithium Carbonate
Magnesium Hydroxide
Magnesium Sulfate
Mannitol
Meperidine Hydrochloride
Methlydopa
Methylphenidate Hydrochloride
Methylprednisolone
Methylprednisolone Acetate
Methylprednisolone Sodium Succinate
Metronidazole
Minoxidil
Morphine Sulfate
Muromonab
Nafcillin Sodium
Naloxone Hydrochloride
Netromycin
Nifedipine
Nitrofurantoin
Nitroprusside Sodium
Oxacillin
Pemoline

Alphabetical Drug Listing

Penicillin V Potassium
Phenobarbital
Phentolamine Mesylate
Phenytoin Sodium
Phytonadione
Potassium Chloride
Prednisone
Primidone
Prochlorperazine
Propranolol Hydrochloride
Rifampin
Sodium Polystyrene Sulfonate
Tetracycline
Theophylline
Ticarcillin Clavulanic Acid
Tobramycin
Trimethoprim Sulfamethoxazole
Valproic Acid
Vancomycin Hydrochloride
Verapamil

Acetaminophen

SYNONYM: Tylenol, Datril, Tempra

CLASS: Analgesic and antipyretic agent (acetaminophen is ***not*** an anti-inflammatory agent)

DOSAGE FORM:
Liquid: 160 mg/5 ml, 320 mg/10 ml, 650 mg/25 ml

Liquid: 120 mg/5 ml with codeine 12 mg/5 ml (Tylenol with codeine elixir)

Suppository: 325 mg, 650 mg

Tablets: (scored) 325 mg

Tablets: 325 mg with codeine 15 mg (Tylenol with codeine No. 2)

Tablets: 325 mg with codeine 30 mg (Tylenol with codeine No. 3)

CONTROLLED SUBSTANCE:
With codeine; Schedule III (C-III)

SELECTED DOSAGES:

Analgesia or Antipyresis: In children >11 years of age: oral or rectal dosage: 325–650 mg every 4–6 hours prn, but less than 4 g daily. For other ages, as follows: oral or rectal doses every 4–6 hours prn: 11 years, 480 mg; 9–10 years, 400 mg, 6–8 years, 320 mg; 4–5 years, 240 mg; 2–3 years, 160 mg; oral doses every 4–6 hours for 1–2 years, 120 mg; 4–11 months, 80 mg; up to 3 months, 40 mg. Rectal doses for <2 years of age must be individualized.

COMMON SIDE EFFECTS: Nontoxic in therapeutic doses.

SELECTED DRUG INTERACTIONS: Possible severe hypothermia in patients receiving phenothiazine and antipyretic therapy.

CAUTIONS: Toxic effects could result from a single toxic dose or from long-term ingestion, leading to dose-dependent hepatic necrosis, which is potentially fatal. Call regional poison control center or the Rocky Mountain Poison Control Center (800–525–6115) for assistance in diagnosis and for directions in the use of acetylcysteine as an antidote. Acetaminophen should not be used for self-medication of pain for longer than 5 days in children unless directed by physician, or for marked fever (>39.5° C) or recurrent fever. No more than 5 doses should be administered to children for analgesia or antipyresis in 24 hours.

Acetazolamide

SYNONYM: Diamox

CLASS: Carbonic anhydrase inhibitor

DOSAGE FORM:
Tablets: (scored) 250 mg

Capsules: prolonged action, 500 mg

Injection: 500 mg

SELECTED DOSAGES:

Glaucoma: Children: oral dosage: 8–30 mg/kg or 300–900 mg/m^2 daily, in 3 divided doses; for *acute glaucoma:* 5–10 mg/kg IM or IV every 6 hours.

Epilepsy: Children: 8–30 mg/kg daily in 1–4 divided doses; initial dose if given with other anticonvulsants: 250 mg.

Diuretic: Children: 5 mg/kg or 150 mg/m^2 orally or IV once daily in AM.

COMMON SIDE EFFECTS: Serious side effects are infrequent, especially with short-term therapy. Most respond to lowering of dosage.

SELECTED DRUG INTERACTIONS: Increases excretion of lithium.

CAUTIONS: Addition, withdrawal, or replacement of an anticonvulsant with another should be done slowly.

Acetohydroxamic Acid

SYNONYM: Lithostat

CLASS: Ammonia detoxicant

DOSAGE FORM: Tablets: (scored) 250 mg

SELECTED DOSAGES: Usual dose and frequency not established in children; manufacturer states initial dosage of 10 mg/kg daily in 2 or 3 divided doses tolerated for up to 1 year in children 8–10 years old.

COMMON SIDE EFFECTS: Adverse effects, including only abnormal laboratory test results in some patients, occur in up to 30% of patients. Commonly seen in patients with renal impairment and during first year of therapy.

SELECTED DRUG INTERACTIONS: Avoid other prescription or over-the-counter drugs, if possible.

CAUTIONS: Close monitoring of child's clinical condition and hematologic status.

Acetylcysteine

SYNONYM: Mucomyst, Mucosol

CLASS: Mucolytic agent

DOSAGE FORM: Solution: 10%, 20%

SELECTED DOSAGES:

Acetaminophen Overdose: Oral or endotracheal loading dose of 140 mg/kg, then 70 mg/kg 4 hours later and every 4 hours for a total of 17 doses. Dilute the 20% solution to a final concentration of 5%.

Direct Nonaerosol Administration by Tracheostomy or Intratracheal Tube: To mobilize thick, tenacious tracheal secretions, use 10% solution, 2–4 ml every 1–4 hours.

COMMON SIDE EFFECTS: Nausea, vomiting, other GI symptoms with oral administration for acetaminophen overdose.

CAUTIONS: Use carefully with asthma patients; discontinue if bronchospasms, which may occur, cannot be treated with nebulizer bronchodilator.

Achromycin: See **tetracycline.**

Acyclovir

SYNONYM: Zovirax

CLASS: Antiviral agent

DOSAGE FORM:
Capsule: 200 mg

Injection: 500 mg vial

Suspension: 200 mg/5 ml

SELECTED DOSAGES:

Mucosal or Cutaneous Herpes Simplex: Parenteral dosage for infections in immunocompromised patients >12 years of age with normal renal function (creatinine clearance >50 ml/min per 1.73 m^2) is 5 mg/kg every 8 hours (15 mg/kg daily) for 7 days; in children <12 years of age, a more accurate dosage is 250 mg/m^2 every 8 hours (750 mg/m^2 daily) for 7 days. Dosages of 5–15 mg/kg or 250 mg/m^2 every 8 hours have been suggested for neonates but should be adjusted according to the maturity of renal function. Reconstitute by adding 10 or 20 ml of sterile water for injection to a 500 mg or 1 g vial, respectively, to providc a solution with 50 mg/ml. The appropriate dose should be withdrawn and further diluted with 50–125 ml of a compatible IV solution. Concentrations of the infusion generally should not exceed 7 mg/ml.

Herpes Simplex Encephalitis: Recommended IV dosage for children >6 months of age is 10 mg/kg every 8 hours (30 mg/kg daily) for 10 days; in children between 6 months and 12 years of age, a more accurate dosage is 500 mg/m^2 every 8 hours (1.5 g/m^2 daily) for 10 days. Because relapses have been reported after only 10 days' treatment, some clinicians recommend a longer duration of treatment (14–21 days). Although the same dosage regimen is currently being evaluated in neonates (not in the approved labeling), some clinicians recommend a neonatal IV dosage of 10 mg/kg every 8 hours (30 mg/kg daily) for 10 days pending availability of more data.

Varicella-Zoster (Chickenpox): In immunocompromised patients the recommended IV dosage for children >12 years of age with normal renal function is 10 mg/kg (infused at a constant rate over 1 hour) every 8 hours (30 mg/kg) for 7 days; in children <12 years of age, equivalent plasma drug concentrations are attained by administering 500 mg/m^2 (infused at a constant rate over 1 hour) every 8 hours (1.5 g/m^2 daily) for 7 days.

COMMON SIDE EFFECTS: Minimal adverse effects with IV administration, but potentially serious reactions (e.g., renal tubular damage) can occur. Follow IV administration rate recommendations carefully.

SELECTED DRUG INTERACTIONS: Refer to manufacturer recommendations when using with zidovudine (AZT), probenecid, antifungal agents, interferon, and methotrexate.

CAUTIONS: Information regarding the use of oral or topical acyclovir in children is lacking or has not been established. ***See manufacturer's recommendations for modification of dose in renal impairment.***

Adalat: See **nifedipine.**

Adrenalin: See **epinephrine.**

Advil: See **ibuprofen.**

Albuterol

SYNONYM: Proventil, Ventolin

CLASS: Sympathomimetic agent; bronchodilator

DOSAGE FORM:
Aerosol: 90 μg/dose, 200 metered doses/inhaler

Liquid: 2 mg/5 ml

Tablets: 2 mg, 4 mg, 4 mg extended release

SELECTED DOSAGES:

Acute Bronchospasm or Prevention of Asthmatic Symptoms: Via metered-dose inhaler, for children >4 years of age: 180 μg (2 inhalations) every 4–6 hours. Via nebulizer, suggested dosages for children ≥12 years of age: 2.5 mg 3 or 4 times daily; for children <5 years of age, 1.25–2.5 mg; or ≥5 years of age, 2.5–5 mg every 4–6 hours. Oral dosage, for children ≥12 years of age: 2 or 4 mg 3 or 4 times daily as tablets or oral solution, or 4 or 8 mg every 12 hours as extended release tablets; for children

6–12 years of age: 2 mg 3 or 4 times daily; for children 2–6 years of age: initial oral dosage 0.1 mg/kg 3 times daily (not to exceed 2 mg 3 times daily) as the oral solution.

COMMON SIDE EFFECTS: Tachycardia, palpitations, peripheral vasodilation, tremor, and nervousness.

SELECTED DRUG INTERACTIONS: Should not be administered with other oral sympathomimetic agents. Monoamine oxidase (MAO) inhibitors or tricyclic antidepressants may potentiate vascular system effects.

CAUTIONS: Many questions about the safety and efficacy of this drug in children have not been answered. The manufacturer's information should be consulted.

Aldomet: See methyldopa.

Amantadine Hydrochloride.

SYNONYM: Symmetrel

CLASS: Antiviral agent, antiparkinsonism agent

DOSAGE FORM:
Capsules: 100 mg

Liquid: 50 mg/5 ml

SELECTED DOSAGES: Influenza A virus infection treatment (200 mg) and prophylaxis (100 or 200 mg) daily for children >10 years of age and with normal renal function. Children 1–9 years of age: 4.4–8.8 mg/kg daily (maximum 150 mg daily) in single dose or two equally divided doses.

COMMON SIDE EFFECTS: Dizziness, insomnia, nervousness, anxiety, and impaired concentration reported in 5–10% of patients.

SELECTED DRUG INTERACTIONS: CNS stimulants, anticholinergic drugs.

CAUTIONS: Safety and efficacy not established for children <1 year of age. Adjust dosage for renal impairment. Use carefully in patients with epilepsy or history of seizures or other CNS disorders.

Amikacin

SYNONYM: Amikin

CLASS: Aminoglycoside

DOSAGE FORM: Injection: 100 mg/2 ml, 500 mg/2 ml

SELECTED DOSAGES: Amikacin sulfate is administered by IM injection or IV infusion. For pediatric patients the volume of infusion fluid depends on the patient's needs but should be sufficient to allow an infusion period of 1–2 hours in infants or 30–60 minutes in older children. The usual dosage recommended by the manufacturer for adults, children, and older infants with normal renal function is 15 mg/kg daily, given in equally divided doses at 8- or 12-hour intervals. Do not exceed 15 mg/kg or 1.5 g. The manufacturer states that safe use of amikacin in neonates and infants has not been established, and the drug should be used in these patients only when other aminoglycosides cannot be used because of bacterial resistance and when the infant can be closely observed for evidence of toxic effects. When amikacin is used in neonates, the manufacturer recommends an initial loading dose of 10 mg/kg followed by 7.5 mg/kg every 12 hours.

COMMON SIDE EFFECTS: Ototoxic and nephrotoxic effects are most serious and can be minimized by proper dosing and careful monitoring.

SELECTED DRUG INTERACTIONS: Neurotoxic, ototoxic, or nephrotoxic drugs, general anesthetics and neuromuscular blocking agents, neomycin, nonsteroidal anti-inflammatory agents.

CAUTIONS: Adjust dosage for renal impairment. Risk of toxic effects may be associated with prolonged peak serum levels >30–35 μg/ml. Trough serum levels should not exceed 5–10 μg/ml.

Amikin: See amikacin.

Amiloride Hydrochloride.

SYNONYM: Moduretic

CLASS: Diuretic

DOSAGE FORM: Tablets: 5 mg: with hydrochlorothiazide, 50 mg

SELECTED DOSAGES: A dosage of 0.625 mg/kg daily has been used in children weighing 6–20 kg.

COMMON SIDE EFFECTS: Similar to those of hydrochlorothiazide. The potassium-sparing effect may cause hyperkalemia.

SELECTED DRUG INTERACTIONS: Avoid using other potassium-sparing diuretics and the concurrent administration of potassium supplements.

CAUTIONS: Safety and efficacy not established in children.

Aminophylline

SYNONYM: Somophyllin-DF

CLASS: Respiratory smooth muscle relaxant

DOSAGE FORM:
Injection: 25 mg (19.7 mg of anhydrous theophylline) per milliliter

Liquid: 105 mg (90 mg of anhydrous theophylline) per 5 ml, dye-free and alcohol-free preparation

Rectal: 250 mg (197.3 mg of anhydrous theophylline)

Tablets: (uncoated) 100 mg (78.9 mg of anhydrous theophylline), 200 mg (157.8 mg of anhydrous theophylline), 225 mg (177.5 mg of anhydrous theophylline)
(Aminophylline contains 80% theophylline by weight.)

SELECTED DOSAGES: Aminophylline, a theophylline compound with ethylenediamine, may be administered undiluted by slow IV injection or, preferably, in large-volume parenteral fluids by slow IV infusion. Avoid IM administration because it causes intense pain. Use the following chart to calculate the dosage of theophylline preparations in terms of anhydrous theophylline. The anhydrous theophylline content in the various theophylline derivatives is approximately:

Drug	Anhydrous Theophylline Content
Aminophylline anhydrous	85.7% (± 1.7%)
Aminophylline hydrous	78.9% (± 1.6%)
Oxitriphylline	63.6% (± 1.9%)
Theophylline monohydrate	90.7% (± 1.1%)

Acute Bronchospasm: For the treatment of acute bronchospasm, theophylline (often as aminophylline) is preferably administered IV. Only the injection containing approximately 20 mg of theophylline (25 mg of aminophylline) per milliliter should be administered IV. To minimize adverse effects, administer IV theophylline slowly, at a rate not exceeding 20 mg/min; loading doses are usually given over 20–30 minutes. If patients have acute adverse effects while loading doses of theophylline are being infused, the infusion may be stopped for 5–10 minutes or administered at a slower rate.

Patients not currently receiving theophylline preparations may receive a theophylline loading dose of 4.7 mg/kg (approximately equivalent to hydrous aminophylline 6 mg/kg) and the following maintenance dosages IV:

Approximate IV Theophylline Dosage for Treatment of Acute Bronchospasm

Group	Maintenance Dosage for Next 12 Hours	Maintenance Dosage After 12 Hours
Children 6 months to 9 years of age	0.95 mg/kg per hour (1.2 mg/kg per hour)*	0.79 mg/kg per hour (1 mg/kg per hour)*
Children 9–16 years of age and young adult smokers	0.79 mg/kg per hour (1 mg/kg per hour)*	0.63 mg/kg per hour (0.8 mg/kg per hour)*

*Equivalent hydrous aminophylline dosage indicated in parentheses.

In patients who are currently receiving theophylline preparations, the time, amount, route of administration, and dosage form of the patient's last dose should be determined when possible and considered in determining a loading dose. Loading doses are based on the general expectation that each 0.5 mg of theophylline per kilogram of lean body weight will result in a 1 μg/ml increase in serum theophylline concentration. Ideally, *in patients who are currently receiving theophylline preparations,* the loading dose should be deferred until a serum theophylline concentration can be attained rapidly; when this is not possible, the clinician must carefully select a dose based on the potential benefits and risks. When there is sufficient respiratory distress in these patients to warrant a small risk, a theophylline loading dose of 2.5 mg/kg may be administered; this dose is likely to increase serum concentrations by about 5 μg/ml and is unlikely to result in dangerous adverse effects if the patient is not currently having a toxic reaction to theophylline. Maintenance dosage should be decreased if adverse effects occur.

Because of the marked variation in theophylline metabolism in children <6 months of age, the manufacturers recommend that theophylline not be administered to these children. However, it has been used in this age group, and specialized references should be consulted for dosage information.

Although IV theophylline is preferred for the treatment of acute bronchospasm, oral solutions or suspensions of the drug or plain, uncoated tablets may also be administered. Other oral dosage forms (e.g., extended-release preparations) should ***not*** be used for acute bronchospasm. *Patients not currently receiving theophylline preparations* may receive a theophylline loading dose of 6 mg/kg and the following maintenance dosages orally:

Approximate Oral Theophylline Dosage for Treatment of Acute Bronchospasm

Group	Dosage for Next 12–16 Hours	Maintenance Dosage
Children 6 months to 9 years of age	4 mg/kg every 4 hours × 3 doses	4 mg/kg every 6 hours
Children 9–16 years of age and young adult smokers	3 mg/kg every 4 hours × 3 doses	3 mg/kg every 6 hours

Chronic Bronchospasm: With rapidly absorbed dosage forms, the usual initial oral dosage of theophylline is 16 mg/kg or 400 mg daily (whichever is less), given in 3 or 4 divided doses at 6- to 8-hour intervals. Although extended-release preparations have been formulated to release the drug at various rates suitable for dosing every 8–12, 12, or 24 hours, the actual dosing frequency for a given patient and preparation depends on the patient's individual pharmacokinetic parameters. When extended-release preparations are administered, the usual initial oral dosage of theophylline in children and adults is 12 mg/kg or 400 mg daily (whichever is less), given in 2 or 3 divided doses at 8- or 12-hour intervals. With rapidly absorbed dosage forms, dosage may be increased, if tolerated, in approximate increments of 25% at 2- to 3-day intervals. With extended-release preparations, dosage may be increased, if tolerated, by 2–3 mg/kg daily at 3-day intervals.

Regardless of dosage form, dosage may be increased, if tolerated, up to the following maximum daily doses, without measurement of serum theophylline concentration:

Children ≤9 years of age	24 mg/kg daily
Children 9–12 years of age	20 mg/kg daily
Patients 12–16 years of age	18 mg/kg daily
Patients ≥16 years of age	13 mg/kg or 900 mg daily (whichever is less)

Dosage adjustments may be based on peak serum theophylline concentrations, and the clinical response and tolerance of the patient are as follows:

Dosage Adjustment After Serum Theophylline Measurement

If Serum Theophylline Level Is	Dosage	Directions
Within normal limits	10–20 μg/ml	Maintain dosage if tolerated; recheck serum theophylline concentration at 6- to 12-month intervals*
Too high	20–25 μg/ml	Decrease doses by about 10%; recheck serum theophylline concentration after 3 days and then at 6- to 12-month intervals*

*Finer adjustments in dosage may be needed in some patients.

Dosage Adjustment After Serum Theophylline Measurement—cont'd

If Serum Theophylline Level Is	Dosage	Directions
Too high	25–30 μg/ml	Skip next dose and decrease subsequent doses by 25%; recheck serum theophylline level
	>30 μg/ml	Skip next 2 doses and decrease subsequent doses by 50%; recheck serum theophylline level
Too low	7.5–10 μg/ml	Increase dose by about 25%†; recheck serum theophylline concentration after 3 days and then at 6- to 12-month intervals*
	5–7.5 μg/ml	Increase dose by about 25% to the nearest dose increment†; recheck serum theophylline level for guidance in further dosage adjustment (another increase will probably be needed, but this provides a safety check)

*Finer adjustments in dosage may be needed for some patients.
†Dividing the daily dose into 3 doses administered at 8-hour intervals may be indicated if symptoms occur repeatedly at the end of a dosing interval.
From Weinberger M, Hendeles L. Practical guide to using theophylline. J Respir Dis 1981;27:12–27.

In children <1 year of age, particularly in premature and term neonates: Dosage has not been well established and must be carefully individualized. Elimination of the drug in children <1 year of age, especially in neonates, generally appears to be reduced. Because of a lack of adequate studies, theophylline is not labeled for use in children <6 months of age. Because of potential toxicity, use of the drug in children <1 year of age should be carefully considered, and if it is used, the initial and maintenance dosages (particularly the latter) should be conservative. The recommended oral or IV loading dose of theophylline in these children is 1 mg/kg for each 2 μg/ml increase in serum concentration desired. The recommended initial maintenance dosage in premature neonates up to 40 weeks of postconceptional age (gestational age at birth plus postnatal age) is 1 mg/kg every 12 hours. The recommended initial maintenance dosage in term neonates (at birth or at 40 weeks of postceptional age) is 1–2 mg/kg every 12 hours in those up to 4 weeks of postnatal age, 1–2 mg/kg every 8 hours in those 4–8 weeks of postnatal age, and 1–3 mg/kg every 6 hours in those >8 weeks of postnatal age. Some clinicians suggest that higher initial and maintenance dosages may be necessary in preterm neonates. The maintenance dosage and the dosing interval must be guided by monitoring serum theophylline concentrations. It is recommended that serum theophylline concentrations be maintained at <10 μg/ml in neonates and 20 μg/ml in older infants. Maintenance dosage should not be exceeded and therapy with the drug should not be continued unless the drug is well tolerated and clinically beneficial.

COMMON SIDE EFFECTS: GI irritation and CNS stimulation, palpitation, tachycardia. Distinguishing symptoms of toxic effects could include frequent vomiting, severe thirst, slight fever, tinnitus, and palpitations. Seizures may occur.

SELECTED DRUG INTERACTIONS: Increase in excretion of lithium; effects of oral anticoagulants may be enhanced.

CAUTIONS: Theophylline has a low therapeutic index; carefully determine dose on the basis of age, weight, and therapeutic serum levels. Normal serum levels are between 10 and 20 μg/ml.

Amitriptyline Hydrochloride

SYNONYM: Elavil, Endep

CLASS: Antidepressant

DOSAGE FORM:
Injection: 10 mg/ml

Tablets: (film coated) 10 mg, 25 mg, 50 mg, 75 mg, 100 mg, 150 mg

SELECTED DOSAGES:

Depression: Safe use of tricyclic antidepressants for the treatment of depression in children <12 years of age is not established.

Chronic Pain: Children: oral: initial: 0.1 mg/kg at bedtime; may advance as tolerated for 2–3 weeks to 0.5–2 mg/kg at bedtime. Adolescents: oral: initial: 25–50 mg/kg; may give in divided doses; increase gradually to 100 mg/day in divided doses. Consult primary literature.

COMMON SIDE EFFECTS: Anticholinergic effects, drowsiness, weakness, lethargy, fatigue.

SELECTED DRUG INTERACTIONS: Monoamine oxidase (MAO) inhibitors; additive depressive effect with other CNS depressants.

CAUTIONS: Severe symptoms or death occur in children who receive >20 mg of imipramine per kilogram.

Amoxicillin

SYNONYM: Polymox, Wymox

CLASS: Penicillin

DOSAGE FORM:
Capsules: 250 mg, 500 mg

Suspension: 125 mg/5 ml, 250 mg/5 ml

SELECTED DOSAGES:

Most Infections Caused by Susceptible Organisms: Children ≥20 kg: usual adult dosage: 250 mg every 8 hours; children <20 kg: doses based on weight. For **severe infections or those caused by less susceptable organisms** a dosage of 500 mg every 8 hours may be needed.

Upper Respiratory Tract Infection, Including Otitis Media: For infants <1 month old and weighing <20 kg: 20 mg/kg daily, given in divided doses every 8 hours; for **severe infections**, 40 mg/kg daily in divided doses every 8 hours.

Lower Respiratory Tract Infections Caused by Susceptible Organisms:: Children ≥20 kg: 500 mg every 8 hours. Children <20 kg: usual dose is 40 mg/kg daily, given in divided doses every 8 hours.

COMMON SIDE EFFECTS: GI, rash, and hypersensitivity reactions.

CAUTIONS: Check for penicillin allergies.

Amoxicillin–Clavulanic Acid

SYNONYM: Augmentin

CLASS: Penicillin

DOSAGE FORM:
Tablets: 250 mg amoxicillin with 125 mg clavulanic acid; 500 mg amoxicillin with 125 mg clavulanic acid

Suspension: 125 mg (amoxicillin) per 5 ml and 31.25 (clavulanic acid) per 5 ml; 250 mg per 5 ml

SELECTED DOSAGES: Dosage of amoxicillin and clavulanate potassium is generally expressed in terms of the amoxicillin content of the fixed combination. For children >40 kg: usual adult oral dose: 250 mg every 8 hours; for severe infections, 500 mg every 8 hours for 7 days. For children <40 kg: 20 mg/kg given in divided doses every 8 hours. Otitis media, sinusitis, lower respiratory tract infections, and severe infections: 40 mg/kg in divided doses every 8 hours.

COMMON SIDE EFFECTS: GI, rash, and hypersensitivity reactions.

CAUTIONS: Check for penicillin allergies.

Ampicillin

SYNONYM: Omnipen, Polycillin

CLASS: Penicillin

DOSAGE FORM:
Tablets: chewable, 125 mg

Capsules: 250 mg, 500 mg

Injection: 250 mg, 500 mg, 1 g, 2 g vials

Suspension: 125 mg/5 ml, 250 mg/5 ml

SELECTED DOSAGES: For oral therapy, most manufacturers state that children weighing >20 kg may receive the usual adult dosage of ampicillin. For parenteral therapy, some manufacturers recommend that the usual adult dosage be given to children weighing >20 kg, whereas other manufacturers and many clinicians recommend that the usual adult dosage be used in those weighing

>40 kg. Pediatric dosage should not exceed dosage recommended for similar infections in adults.

Respiratory Tract or Skin and Skin Structure Infections: Usual dosage for children weighing ≤40 kg: 25–50 mg/kg daily, administered in equally divided doses every 6 hours.

GI or Urinary Tract Infections: Usual dosage for children weighing ≤ 40 kg: 50–100 mg/kg daily, given in equally divided doses every 6 hours.

Septicemia or CNS Infections: Usual pediatric dosage recommended by manufacturers: 100–200 mg/kg daily, given in divided doses every 3–4 hours, starting with IV administration for 3 days and continuing with IM administration. Alternatively, many clinicians recommend that children >1 month of age receive dosages of 50–100 mg/kg daily, given orally, IM, or IV in divided doses every 6–8 hours for the treatment of mild to moderate infections, and 200–400 mg/kg daily, given IM or IV in divided doses every 4–6 hours for the treatment of severe infections. Some clinicians suggest a maximum dosage of 12 g daily in children. Many clinicians recommend that neonates ≤1 week old receive a dosage of 25 mg/kg IM or IV every 12 hours (for those ≤2 kg) or 8 hours (for those >2 kg), and that neonates >1 week of age receive this dose IM or IV every 8 hours (for those ≤2 kg) or every 6 hours (for those >2 kg) for the treatment of infections other than meningitis.

Bacterial Meningitis: For empiric treatment of neonates and children <2 months of age, many clinicians recommend that an IV ampicillin dosage of 100–300 mg/kg daily be given in divided doses in conjunction with IM gentamicin pending results of in vitro susceptibility tests.

Neonatal Meningitis Caused by Susceptible Organisms: Most clinicians recommend that neonates ≤1 week of age receive an IV dosage of 50–75 mg/kg every 12 hours (for those ≤2 kg) or every 8 hours (for those >2 kg) and that neonates >1 week of age receive 50 mg/kg IV every 8 hours (for those ≤2 kg) or 6 hours (for those >2 kg).

Bacterial Meningitis: For empiric treatment of children 2 months to 12 years of age, many clinicians recommend that an IV dosage of 200–400 mg/kg daily be given in divided doses every 4–6 hours in conjunction with IV chloramphenicol. If bacterial susceptibility data are not available and clinical and bacteriologic response is unsatisfactory after 24–48 hours, other appropriate anti-infective therapy should be substituted.

Life-threatening Septicemia: For initial therapy in neonates, ampicillin has been administered IM in conjunction with an aminoglycoside (e.g., gentamicin). Term and preterm neonates <7 days of age: 50 mg/kg daily in equally divided doses every 12 hours. Preterm neonates 7–28 days of age: 100 mg/kg daily in equally divided doses every 8 hours. Term neonates 7–28 days of age: 150 mg/kg daily in equally divided doses every 8 hours.

COMMON SIDE EFFECTS: Diarrhea and rash.

SELECTED DRUG INTERACTIONS: Rare; may mimic those seen with penicillin G.

CAUTIONS: Check for penicillin allergies.

Amrinone Lactate

SYNONYM: Inocor

CLASS: Cardiac drug

DOSAGE FORM: Injection: 5 mg/ml (do not dilute in dextrose-containing solutions)

SELECTED DOSAGES: A few children ≥12 years of age have received amrinone for severe congestive heart failure. Dosage should not exceed 10 mg/kg per 24 hours. Neonates: 0.75 mg/kg IV bolus for 2–3 minutes, followed by maintenance infusion of 3–5 μg/kg/minute; IV bolus may need to be repeated in 30 minutes. Children 0.75 mg/kg IV bolus for 2–3 minutes, followed by maintenance infusion 5–10 μg/kg per minute; IV bolus may need to be repeated in 30 minutes.

COMMON SIDE EFFECTS: Thrombocytopenia has occurred in 2.4% of patients given short-term therapy and usual doses.

SELECTED DRUG INTERACTIONS: Extensive hypotension with disopyramide.

CAUTIONS: Safety and efficacy in children <18 years of age not established.

Anafranil: See **clomipramine.**

Apresoline: See **hydralazine.**

Ascriptin: See **aspirin.**

Aspirin

SYNONYM: Ascriptin, Bayer Children's, Ecotrin, Empirin with Codeine

CLASS: Analgesic and antipyretic agent

DOSAGE FORM:
Suppositories: 65 mg, 325 mg, 650 mg

Tablets: 65 mg (children's), 81 mg, (scored) 325 mg

Tablets: (buffered) 325 mg (Bufferin)

Tablets: (enteric coated) 325 mg (Ecotrin)

Tablets: 325 mg with codeine 15 mg (aspirin with codeine No. 2)

Tablets: 325 mg with codeine 30 mg (aspirin with codeine No. 3)

CONTROLLED SUBSTANCE: With codeine: Schedule III DEA (C-III)

SELECTED DOSAGES:

Analgesia/Antipyresis: Children >11 years of age: usual oral or rectal dose: 325–650 mg every 4 hours; do not exceed 4 g daily. Children 2–11 years of age: oral or rectal dose: 1.5 g/m^2 daily or 65 mg/kg daily, in 4–6 divided doses; total rectal dose no more than 2.5 g/m^2. General doses every 4 hours, oral or rectal administration: children 11 years of age: 480 mg; 9–12 years, 400 mg; 6–8 years, 325 mg; 4–5 years, 240 mg; 2–3 years, 160 mg. Children <2 years of age: individual dosage. Refer to manufacturer's information for different dosage forms of aspirin (e.g., gum, buffered). ***Administer with full glass of water or milk to reduce GI irritation.***

COMMON SIDE EFFECTS: GI irritation: dyspepsia, nausea.

SELECTED DRUG INTERACTIONS: Most important: anticoagulants and thrombolytic agents, sulfonylureas, corticosteroids, methotrexate.

CAUTIONS: Use carefully in children who are dehydrated, because they are susceptible to salicylate toxicity. The U.S. Surgeon General, the American Academy of Pediatrics Committee on Infectious Diseases, the U.S. Food and Drug Administration (FDA), and others advise that salicylates should not be used in children and teenagers with varicella or influenza unless directed by a physician.

Atarax: See **hydroxyzine.**

Atenolol

SYNONYM: Tenormin

CLASS: Cardiac drug

DOSAGE FORM: Tablets: (scored) 25 mg, 50 mg, 100 mg

SELECTED DOSAGES: Consult the literature for use in children. Usual dose: oral: 1–2 mg/kg per dose, given daily.

COMMON SIDE EFFECTS: Bradycardia in 3% of patients, profound hypotension, coldness of extremities in up to 12%, postural hypotension in 2–4%, dizziness, fatigue.

SELECTED DRUG INTERACTIONS: Use with reserpine may increase incidence of hypotension and bradycardia.

CAUTIONS: Safety and efficacy not established in children. Avoid abrupt withdrawal of drug.

Augmentin: See **amoxicillin–clavulanic acid.**

Azathioprine

SYNONYM: Imuran

CLASS: Unclassified therapeutic agent

DOSAGE FORM:
Tablets: (scored) 50 mg

Injection: 100 mg

SELECTED DOSAGES: 3–5 mg/kg daily, starting on the day of (some cases 1–3 days before) transplantation. After transplant, may be given IV in same dose until oral therapy can be tolerated (usually 1–4 days). When severe hematologic or other toxic effects occur, drug should be discontinued.

COMMON SIDE EFFECTS: Bone marrow suppression: leukopenia, macrocytic anemia, pancytopenia, thrombocytopenia, prolongation of clotting time, and hemorrhage; give dose in divided doses with or after meals.

SELECTED DRUG INTERACTIONS: Reduce dose of azathioprine by 25–33% *if given with allopurinol.*

CAUTIONS: Reduce dose if given with allopurinol or if renal function is impaired.

Bactrim: See **trimethoprim-sulfamethoxazole.**

Benadryl: See **diphenhydramine hydrochloride.**

Bentyl: See **dicyclomine hydrochloride.**

Calan: See **verapamil.**

Capoten: See **captopril.**

Captopril

SYNONYM: Capoten

CLASS: Cardiac drug

DOSAGE FORM: Tablets: (scored) 12.5 mg, 25 mg, 50 mg, 100 mg (may exhibit a sulfurous odor)

SELECTED DOSAGES: Consult literature for dosage listed. Dosage must be titrated according to the patient's response. Neonates: initial: 0.05–0.1 mg/kg per dose, given every 6–24 hours. Infants: initial: 0.15–0.3 mg/kg per dose; titrate dose upward to maximum of 6 mg/kg per day in 1–4 divided doses; usual required dose: 2.5–6 mg/kg per day. Children: initial: 0.5 mg/kg per dose; titrate upward to maximum of 6 mg/kg per day in 2–4 divided doses. Older children: initial: 6.25–12.5 mg/dose every 12–24 hours; titrate to maximum of 6 mg/kg day. Adolescents and adults: initial: 12.5–25 mg/dose given every 8–12 hours; increase by 25 mg/dose to maximum of 450 mg/day.

COMMON SIDE EFFECTS: Rash; loss of taste perception. Side effects leading to discontinuance of therapy have been reported in 4–12% of patients.

SELECTED DRUG INTERACTIONS: Digoxin serum levels may increase by 15–30%; additive effects with diuretics; small increases in serum potassium concentration are seen.

CAUTIONS: Safety and efficacy in children not established; however, there is some clinical experience in children 2 months to 15 years old with secondary hypertension and varying degrees of renal impairment.

Carbamazepine

SYNONYM: Tegretol

CLASS: Anticonvulsants

DOSAGE FORM:
Suspension: 100 mg/5 ml

Tablets: 200 mg

SELECTED DOSAGES: Adjust dosage carefully. Oral suspension: 50 mg 4 times daily in children 6–12 years of age; increase slowly. When converting from tablets to oral suspension, administer total dose in smaller and more frequent doses (e.g., from every 12 to every 8 hours or 3 times a day).

Seizures: Children >12 years of age: 200 mg twice daily (tablets) or 100 mg 4 times daily as suspension. Children 6–12 years of age: 100 mg twice daily (tablets) or 50 mg 4 times a day as suspension.

COMMON SIDE EFFECTS: Transient or persistent minor hematologic changes; leukopenia, agranulocytosis, thrombocytopenia, bone marrow suppression, and cardiovascular, hepatic, and renal disturbances have been reported.

SELECTED DRUG INTERACTIONS: Monitor serum concentrations of other anticonvulsants and adjust doses as necessary because carbamazepine may cause reductions in the serum level of these drugs.

CAUTIONS: Safety and efficacy not established in children <6 years of age.

Catapres: See **clonidine hydrochloride.**

Ceclor: See **cefaclor.**

Cefaclor

SYNONYM: Ceclor

CLASS: Cephalosporin

DOSAGE FORM:
Capsules: 250 mg, 500 mg

Suspension: 125 mg, 187 mg, 250 mg, 375 mg per 5 ml

SELECTED DOSAGES: Children ≥1 month of age: 20 mg/kg daily given in divided doses every 8 hours

Severe Infections, Otitis Media, or Infections with Less Susceptible Organisms: 40 mg/kg daily; maximum daily dose, 1 g.

COMMON SIDE EFFECTS: Hypersensitivity reactions (e.g., urticaria, pruritus, rash, fever and chills) reported in 5% of patients. Nausea, vomiting, and diarrhea are also common.

SELECTED DRUG INTERACTIONS: Concurrent use of nephrotoxic drugs such as the aminoglycosides should be avoided, if possible, because the risk of nephrotoxic effects may be increased.

CAUTIONS: Safety and efficacy in children <1 month of age not established. Conduct patient history of reactions to cephalosporins, penicillins, and other drugs. Do not use if there is a history of reactions to cephalosporins.

Cefixime

SYNONYM: Suprax

CLASS: Cephalosporin

DOSAGE FORM:
Capsules: 200 mg, 400 mg

Suspension: 100 mg per 5 ml

SELECTED DOSAGES: Children >12 years of age or weighing >50 kg may receive the usual adult dosage of cefixime. The usual dosage for children 6 months to 12 years of age is 8 mg/kg daily. This dosage may be given as a single daily dose, or 4 mg/kg may be given every 12 hours. Treatment duration varies from 7–14 days for most indications.

COMMON SIDE EFFECTS: Adverse effects are similar to other cephalosporins. Generally well tolerated; yet adverse effects have been reported in up to 50% of patients but have been severe enough to cause only discontinuation of the drug in 2–4% of patients. Diarrhea, abdominal pain, nausea, anorexia, vomiting, dyspepsia.

SELECTED DRUG INTERACTIONS: Concurrent use of nephrotoxic drugs such as the aminoglycosides should be avoided if possible because the risk of nephrotoxic effects may be increased. Antacids, probenecid, salicylates.

CAUTIONS: Safety and efficacy of cefixime in children <6 months of age not established. The incidence of adverse GI effects, including diarrhea and loose stools, in children receiving cefixime oral suspension reportedly is comparable to that reported in adults receiving tablets of the drug. Diarrhea or loose stools have been reported in up to 15% of children 6 months to 13 years of age receiving oral cefixime. Inquire about previous hypersensitivity reactions to penicillins, cephalosporins, or other drugs.

Cefotaxime

SYNONYM: Claforan

CLASS: Cephalosporin

DOSAGE FORM: Injection: 500 mg, 1 g, 2 g vial

SELECTED DOSAGES: Usual dosage: preterm or term neonates <1 week of age: 50 mg/kg every 12 hours; neonates 1–4 weeks of age: 50 mg/kg every 6–8 hours; children 1 month to 12 years of age and <50 kg: 50–180 mg/kg daily, given in 4–6 equally divided doses; children ≥50 kg: usual daily adult dosage, not to exceed 12 g daily.

Gonococcal Ophthalmia or Disseminated Gonococcal Infection (not included in FDA labeling): Neonates and infants: usual dosage: 25 mg/kg every 8–12 hours for 7 days.

Gonococcal Meningitis: Neonates and infants: 25–50 mg/kg every 8–12 hours for 10–14 days (recommended by many clinicians; also not in manufacturer labeling).

Documented Gonococcal Infection at Any Site (e.g., the eye): Neonates and infants should be evaluated for the possibility of disseminated infection. If disseminated gonococcal infection is present, the Centers for Disease Control and Prevention (CDC) currently recommends 7 days (14 days for meningitis) of therapy with cefotaxime or an equivalent third-generation cephalosporin. Duration of therapy should be for at least 48–72 hours after patient becomes afebrile or there is evidence of eradication of the infection.

COMMON SIDE EFFECTS: Local reactions at injection site, anorexia, diarrhea, nausea, vomiting, abdominal pain.

SELECTED DRUG INTERACTIONS: Concurrent use of nephrotoxic drugs such as the aminoglycosides should be avoided if possible because the risk of nephrotoxic effects may be increased.

CAUTIONS: Conduct patient history of reactions to cephalosporins, penicillins, and other drugs. Do not use if there is a history of reactions to cephalosporins.

Ceftazidime

SYNONYM: Fortaz, Tazicef, Tazidime

CLASS: Cephalosporin

DOSAGE FORM: Injection: 500 mg, 1 g, 2 g vial (either with sodium bicarbonate or arginine)

SELECTED DOSAGES: Arginine formulation for use in children >12 years of age who can receive usual adult dose: 1 g IV or IM every 8 or 12 hours.

Severe Infections: 2 g IV every 8 hours. Children 1 month to 12 years of age: 30–50 mg/kg IV every 8 hours (maximum dose 6 g daily). Immunocompromised patients or patients with cystic fibrosis or meningitis: 50 mg/kg every 8 hours. Neonates ≤4 weeks old: 30 mg/kg every 12 hours.

COMMON SIDE EFFECTS: Adverse effects have been reported in 9% of patients, leading to discontinuance in 2%. Eosinophilia in 7%, thrombocytosis in about 2% of patients. Nausea, vomiting, diarrhea.

SELECTED DRUG INTERACTIONS: Concurrent use of nephrotoxic drugs such as the aminoglycosides should be avoided if possible because the risk of nephrotoxic effects may be increased.

CAUTIONS: Conduct patient history of reactions to cephalosporins, penicillins, and other drugs. Do not use if there is a history of reactions to cephalosporins.

Ceftriaxone

SYNONYM: Rocephin

CLASS: Cephalosporin

DOSAGE FORM: Injection: 250 mg, 1 g, 2 g vials

SELECTED DOSAGES: Children >12 years of age: usual adult dose: 1–2 g once daily or in equally divided doses twice daily.

Serious Infections (Not Including Meningitis): Neonates and children ≤12 years of age: 50–75 mg/kg daily in equally divided doses every 12 hours.

CNS Infections: Neonates and children ≤12 years of age: 100 mg/kg daily in equally divided doses every 12 hours; a 75 mg/kg loading dose may be used to start therapy. Consult manufacturer literature for other dosage recommendations.

COMMON SIDE EFFECTS: Adverse effects have been reported in 10% of patients, leading to discontinuance in 2%. Eosinophilia in 6%, thrombocytosis in about 5% of patients. Nausea, vomiting, diarrhea.

CAUTIONS: Conduct patient history of reactions to cephalosporins, penicillins, and other drugs. Do not use if there is a history of reactions to cephalosporins. Do not administer to neonates with hyperbilirubinemia, particularly premature neonates, because drug can displace bilirubin from serum albumin. Do not reconstitute IM form with bacteriostatic diluent containing benzyl alcohol.

Cephalexin

SYNONYM: Cefanex, Keflex, Keftab

CLASS: Cephalosporin

DOSAGE FORM:

Capsules: 250 mg, 500 mg

Suspension: 125 mg/5 ml, 250 mg/5 ml, 100 mg/ml (pediatric drops)

SELECTED DOSAGES: Usual dosage for children: 25–50 mg/kg daily. For severe infections, these dosages may be doubled. Although the daily dosage is usually administered in 4 equally divided doses, the manufacturers state that daily dosage may be given in 2 equally divided doses at 12-hour intervals for the treatment of streptococcal pharyngitis in patients >1 year of age or for the treatment of skin and skin structure infections in children. Alternatively, some clinicians recommend a pediatric dosage of 0.75–1.5 g/m^2 daily, administered in 4 equally divided doses. For the treatment of otitis media, the manufacturers recommend a pediatric dosage of 75–100 mg/kg daily in 4 divided doses.

COMMON SIDE EFFECTS: Hypersensitivity reactions (e.g., urticaria, pruritus, rash, fever, and chills) reported in 5% of patients. Nausea, vomiting, diarrhea.

SELECTED DRUG INTERACTIONS: Concurrent use of nephrotoxic drugs such as the aminoglycosides should be avoided if possible because the risk of nephrotoxic effects may be increased.

CAUTIONS: Conduct patient history of reactions to cephalosporins, penicillins, and other drugs. Do not use if there is a history of reactions to cephalosporins.

Cephalothin

SYNONYM: Keflin

CLASS: Cephalosporin

DOSAGE FORM: Injection: 1 g, 2 g

SELECTED DOSAGES: Usual dose: 80–160 mg/kg daily in divided doses, or 3 g/m^2 daily in 4 equally divided doses. Perioperative prophylaxis: 20–30 mg/kg 30–60 minutes before surgery and every 6 hours postoperatively. For ventriculitis in children with hydroencephaly: 15–100 mg daily intraventricularly or via a ventricular shunt.

COMMON SIDE EFFECTS: Hypersensitivity reactions (e.g., urticaria, pruritus, rash, fever and chills) reported in 5% of patients. Nausea, vomiting, diarrhea.

SELECTED DRUG INTERACTIONS: Concurrent use of nephrotoxic drugs such as the aminoglycosides should be avoided if possible because the risk of nephrotoxic effects may be increased.

CAUTIONS: Conduct patient history of reactions to cephalosporins, penicillins, and other drugs. Do not use if there is a history of reactions to cephalosporins.

Chlorothiazide

SYNONYM: Diuril

CLASS: Diuretic

DOSAGE FORM:
Suspension: 250 mg/5 ml

Tablets: 250 mg, 500 mg

SELECTED DOSAGES: Children 6 months to 12 years of age: 20–22 mg/kg or 600 mg/m² daily in 2 divided doses. Infants <6 months of age may require up to 33 mg/kg daily in 2 divided doses. Dose may range from 375 mg to 1 g in children 2–12 years of age and 125 mg–375 mg in children up to 2 years of age.

COMMON SIDE EFFECTS: Potassium depletion; other side effects, other than electrolyte and metabolic disturbances, are rare.

SELECTED DRUG INTERACTIONS: Toxic reaction to digitalis may occur with concurrent administration of diuretics; reduction of lithium elimination may lead to toxic reaction.

CAUTIONS: IV administration in children is limited and is not recommended.

Cipro: See **ciprofloxacin.**

Ciprofloxacin

SYNONYM: Cipro

CLASS: Quinolone

DOSAGE FORM:
Injection: 200 mg, 400 mg

Tablets: 250 mg, 500 mg, 750 mg

SELECTED DOSAGES: Usual adult dosage for mild to moderate infection of lower respiratory tract, skin and skin structure, or bones and joints: 500 mg every 12 hours; consult the primary literature for doses used in pediatric patients.

COMMON SIDE EFFECTS: Reported in 5–14% of patients, resulting in discontinuance in 2–3.5% of patients. GI tract or CNS effects most frequent.

SELECTED DRUG INTERACTIONS: Antacids can cause 14–50% reductions in serum ciprofloxacin concentrations. Coumarin anticoagulants, xanthine derivatives.

CAUTIONS: Drug causes arthropathy in immature animals, and the manufacturer states that the drug should not be used in children. Some clinicians state that it should not be used in children <16–18 years of age, although other clinicians suggest that quinolones may be used cautiously in adolescents if skeletal growth is complete. Some clinicians also suggest that the potential benefits may outweigh the possible risks in certain children 9–18 years of age with serious infections (e.g., patients with cystic fibrosis) when the causative organism is resistant to other available anti-infective agents. Ciprofloxacin has been used in a limited number of children with cystic fibrosis, but transient arthropathy has occurred occasionally in such children.

Claforan: See **cefotaxime.**

Clomipramine

SYNONYM: Anafranil

CLASS: Antidepressant

DOSAGE FORM: Capsules: 25 mg, 50 mg

SELECTED DOSAGES: Safety and effectiveness in children <10 years of age not established.

Initial Treatment and Dosage Adjustment: Children and adolescents: as with adults, the starting dose is 25 mg daily and should be gradually increased (also given in divided doses with meals to reduce gastrointestinal side effects) during the first 2 weeks as tolerated, up to a daily maximum of 3 mg/kg or 100 mg, whichever is smaller. Thereafter the dosage may be increased gradually during the next several weeks up to a daily maximum of 3 mg/kg or 200 mg, whichever is smaller. As with adults, after titration the total daily dose may be given at bedtime to minimize daytime sedation.

Maintenance and Continuation of Treatment: Efficacy after 10 weeks has not been documented in controlled trials; yet patients have been treated for up to 1 year without loss of benefit. Dosage adjustments should be made to maintain patient on lowest effective dosage. Total daily dosage may be given at bedtime.

COMMON SIDE EFFECTS: Gastrointestinal complaints, dry mouth, constipation, nausea, anorexia, somnolence, tremor, dizziness, fatigue, tachycardia, sexual dysfunction, weight gain.

SELECTED DRUG INTERACTIONS: Other CNS-active drugs. Should not be used with monoamine oxidase (MAO) inhibitors, warfarin, digoxin.

CAUTIONS: Should not be given in combination, or 14 days before or after treatment, with an MAO inhibitor. Hyperpyretic crisis, seizures, coma, and death have been reported. To reduce the potential for seizures occurring with the use of the drug, prescribers are advised to limit the daily dose to a maximum of 3 mg/kg (200 mg) in children and adolescents. Take suicide precautions (if treating obsessive-compulsive disorder) by prescribing small quantities to reduce the risk of overdose.

Clonidine Hydrochloride

SYNONYM: Catapres, Catapres-TTS

CLASS: Hypotensive agent

DOSAGE FORM:

Tablets: (scored) 0.1 mg, 0.2 mg, 0.3 mg

Transdermal patch: 0.1 mg, 0.2 mg, 0.3 mg

SELECTED DOSAGES: Consult primary literature for pediatric doses used by clinicians. Children: initial: 5–10 μg/kg per day in divided doses every 8–12 hours; increase gradually to 5–25 μg/kg per day in divided doses every 6 hours; maximum: 0.9 mg/day.

COMMON SIDE EFFECTS: Dry mouth, drowsiness and sedation, constipation. Dizziness, headache, fatigue, and weakness.

SELECTED DRUG INTERACTIONS: May potentiate the action of other CNS depressant drugs such as opiates or other analgesics or sedatives.

CAUTIONS: Safe use of oral form for hypertension in children not established, but studies are under way to determine safety and efficacy. Safety and efficacy of transdermal form in children <12 years of age not established.

Codeine Phosphate

CLASS: Analgesic and antipyretic agent; expectorant and cough preparation

DOSAGE FORM:
Elixir: 10 mg/5 ml with terpin hydrate 85 mg

Injection: 30 mg/ml, 60 mg/ml

Syrup: 11 mg/5 ml with expectorant

CONTROLLED SUBSTANCE: Schedule II (C-II); Cheracol with alcohol and codeine: schedule V (C-V)

SELECTED DOSAGES:

Analgesia: Children may receive 3 mg/kg or 100 mg/m^2 daily in 6 divided doses orally, subcutaneously, or IM. Children may also be given 0.5 mg/kg or 15 mg/m^2 every 4–6 hours.

COMMON SIDE EFFECTS: GI effects: nausea, vomiting, constipation.

SELECTED DRUG INTERACTIONS: Other sedative or depressant drugs will potentiate sedation.

CAUTIONS: Respiratory depression and, to a lesser degree, circulatory depression are chief hazards of therapy. Avoid rapid IV administration.

Compazine: See **prochlorperazine.**

Co-Trimoxazole: See **trimethoprim-sulfamethoxazole.**

CTX: See **cyclophosphamide.**

Cyclophosphamide

SYNONYM: CTX, Cytoxan, Neosar

CLASS: Antineoplastic agent

DOSAGE FORM:
Injection: 100 mg, 200 mg, 500 mg, 1 g, 2 g vials

Tablets: 25 mg, 50 mg

SELECTED DOSAGES: Pediatric induction doses: 2–8 mg/kg or 60–250 mg/m^2 daily orally or IV. Recommended maintenance doses: 2–5 mg/kg orally or 50–150 mg/m^2 orally, administered twice weekly.

COMMON SIDE EFFECTS: Leukopenia an expected effect; may be severe, occurring at 8–15 days after single dose, with recovery usually within 17–28 days. Anorexia, nausea, vomiting. Alopecia common.

SELECTED DRUG INTERACTIONS: Barbiturates and other drugs that induce liver microsomal enzymes may increase effect and toxicity of cyclophosphamide.

CAUTIONS: Hematologic toxic effects are major dose-limiting effects. Sterile hemorrhagic cystitis reported to occur in up to 20% of patients, especially children receiving long-term therapy. Observe hydration protocol to reduce adverse effects. Maintain leukocyte count at a range of 2500–4000/mm^3.

Cylert: See **pemoline.**

Cytoxan: See **cyclophosphamide.**

Datril: See **acetaminophen.**

Deltasone: See **prednisone.**

Demerol: See **meperidine hydrochloride.**

Depakene: See valproic acid.

Depo-Medrol: See methylprednisolone.

Desipramine Hydrochloride.

SYNONYM: Norpramin, Pertofrane

CLASS: Psychotherapeutic drug, antidepressant

DOSAGE FORM: Tablets: 10 mg, 25 mg, 50 mg, 75 mg, 100 mg, 150 mg

SELECTED DOSAGES: Safe use of tricyclic antidepressants for depression in children <12 years of age not established.

COMMON SIDE EFFECTS: Anticholinergic effects: dry mucous membranes, blurred vision, constipation.

SELECTED DRUG INTERACTIONS: Monoamine oxidase (MAO) inhibitors, hypotensive agents, CNS depressants.

CAUTIONS: Abrupt withdrawal after prolonged therapy with high doses may cause syndrome with anxiety, chills, headache, dizziness.

Dexedrine: See dextroamphetamine sulfate.

Dextroamphetamine Sulfate

SYNONYM: Dexedrine

CLASS: Respiratory and cerebral stimulant

DOSAGE FORM:
Capsules: Prolonged action, 10 mg

Tablets: 5 mg

CONTROLLED SUBSTANCE: Schedule II (C-II)

SELECTED DOSAGES:

Narcolepsy: Children ≥12 years of age: initial dose: 10 mg daily; increased by 10 mg daily each week until optimal response. Children 6–12 years of age: 5 mg daily, increased by 5 mg each week to response.

Attention Deficit Disorder: Children ≤6 years of age: 5 mg once or twice daily, increased by 5 mg each week to response. Children 3–5 years of age: initial daily dose: 2.5 mg, increased by 2.5 mg each week to response. Give initial dose on awakening. If given in divided doses (2 or 3), additional doses are given at 4- to 6-hour intervals.

COMMON SIDE EFFECTS: Nervousness, insomnia, irritability, dizziness, headaches, blurred vision, hyperexcitability.

SELECTED DRUG INTERACTIONS: Other drugs that produce a hyperexcitability state, monoamine oxidase (MAO) inhibitor drugs.

CAUTIONS: Avoid using as anorectic agent in children <12 years of age. Long-term use in children may suppress weight and/or height patterns. Reduce dosage when intolerable effects, such as anorexia or insomnia, occur. Consult manufacturer information on amphetamines before prescribing. Prolonged use may lead to habituation and possibly to physical or psychic dependence.

Diamox: See **acetazolamide.**

Diazepam

SYNONYM: Valium

CLASS: Benzodiazepine

DOSAGE FORM:
Solution: 5 mg/5 ml, concentrate 5 mg/ml

Tablets: 2 mg, 5 mg, 10 mg

Injection: 5 mg/ml

SELECTED DOSAGES:

Oral: Children >6 months of age: initial oral dosage may be

1–2.5 mg 3 or 4 times daily as conventional tablets or oral solution. Alternatively, some clinicians recommend 0.12–0.8 mg/kg or 3.5–24 mg/m^2 orally in 3 or 4 divided doses daily as conventional tablets. Dosage is adjusted gradually according to response and tolerance. As an adjunct in the *management of epilepsy* in children, a dosage of 6–15 mg daily (and occasionally up to 30 mg daily), in divided doses as conventional tablets or oral solution, has been used by some clinicians. The administration of 15 mg of oral diazepam once daily as extended-release capsules in children >6 months of age is recommended only when it has been determined that the optimal dosage is 5 mg 3 times daily as conventional tablets or oral solution.

Parenteral: In children, IV diazepam should be given slowly during a 3-minute period. The manufacturers recommend that the initial dose not exceed 0.25 mg/kg; the dose may be repeated at 15- to 30-minute intervals to a maximum total of 0.75 mg/kg. For the *management of seizures* in children 30 days to 5 years of age, the usual initial IV dose of diazepam is 0.2–0.5 mg; this dose may be repeated every 2–5 minutes until a maximum total of 5 mg has been given. In children ≥5 years of age, the initial IV dose for the management of seizures is 1 mg; this dose may be repeated every 2–5 minutes until a maximum total of 10 mg has been given. Diazepam may have a short duration of action after IV administration, and it may be necessary to readminister the drug. After seizures are terminated, appropriate *maintenance anticonvulsant therapy* should be instituted. If necessary, the initial dose may be repeated in 2–4 hours. Diazepam may be given IM if seizures make IV administration impossible. For tetanus in children, the manufacturers recommend 1–2 mg for infants >30 days to 5 years of age and 5–10 mg for children >5 years of age administered slowly IV. This dose may be repeated every 3–4 hours as needed. In *painful musculoskeletal conditions and spasticity including tetanus* in children, some clinicians recommend 0.04–0.3 mg/kg IV every 2–4 hours; however, the dosage generally should not exceed 0.6 mg/kg in an 8-hour period. Although the manufacturers have not established pediatric dosage recommendations for *preoperative sedation*, some clinicians have recommended IM administration of 0.4 mg/kg in children older than 2 years of age 1–2 hours before surgery. For *acute anxiety reactions* in children, some clinicians recommend 0.04–0.2 mg/kg IV; this dose may be repeated in 3–4 hours, but dosage should not exceed 0.6 mg/kg in an 8-hour period. Although the safety and efficacy of parenteral diazepam in infants ≤30 days of age have not been established, neonates with agitation caused by opiate withdrawal have received 0.5–2 mg IM every 8 hours followed by gradual reduction in dosage.

COMMON SIDE EFFECTS: Dose-dependent adverse CNS effects are common; they include drowsiness, ataxia, fatigue, confusion, weakness, dizziness, vertigo, and syncope.

SELECTED DRUG INTERACTIONS: CNS depressants, disulfiram, cimetidine, anticonvulsants, psychotherapeutic agents, antacids.

CAUTIONS: Safety and efficacy of oral diazepam in infants <6 months of age not established. Safety and efficacy or parenteral diazepam in infants ≤30 days of age not established.

Diazoxide

SYNONYM: Hyperstat

CLASS: Hypotensive agent

DOSAGE FORM: Injection: 15 mg/ml

SELECTED DOSAGES: Dosage of IV diazoxide for the management of severe hypertension must be adjusted according to the degree of hypertension and the patient's blood pressure response and tolerance.

Severe Hypertension: In children, it is now recommended that diazoxide be administered in doses of 1–3 mg/kg IV every 5–15 minutes until adequate effect is achieved.

Hypoglycemia: Children: initial dose: 3 mg/kg daily divided into 3 equal doses given every 8 hours. Maintenance dose: 3–8 mg/kg daily in 2 or 3 divided doses at 8- or 12-hour intervals. Neonates and infants: initial dose: 10 mg/kg daily, divided in 3 equal doses given every 8 hours; maintenance dose: 8–15 mg/kg per day, divided in 2 or 3 equal doses and given every 12 or 8 hours, respectively.

COMMON SIDE EFFECTS: Hypotension, nausea and vomiting, dizziness, weakness.

SELECTED DRUG INTERACTIONS: Concurrent diuretics may cause increased effect, other hypotensive drugs will be additive effect.

CAUTIONS: Overdosage produces hyperglycemia and possibly ketoacidosis, which should be treated promptly with insulin and restoration of fluid and electrolyte balance.

Dicyclomine Hydrochloride

SYNONYM: Bentyl

CLASS: Anticholinergic antimuscarinic-antispasmodic

DOSAGE FORM:
Capsules: 10 mg

Liquid: oral, 10 mg/5 ml

SELECTED DOSAGES: Consult literature; safety in children not established. Infants >6 months of age: 5 mg/dose 3–4 times daily. Children: 10 mg/dose 3–4 times daily.

COMMON SIDE EFFECTS: Antimuscarinic effects: dry mouth, blurred vision, cycloplegia, mydriasis, tachycardia, palpitation, and constipation.

CAUTIONS: Should be used with caution in infants because of some reports of respiratory distress, seizures, asphyxia, and coma in children ≤6 weeks of age who received dicyclomine orally. Manufacturer of Bentyl states that dicyclomine is contraindicated for use in infants <6 months of age.

Digoxin

SYNONYM: Lanoxin

CLASS: Cardiac drug

DOSAGE FORM:
Capsules, liquid-filled: 50 μg, 100 μg, 200 μg

Tablets, scored: 125 μg; not scored: 250 μg, 500 μg

Elixir: oral, 50 μg/ml

Injection: 10 μg/ml, 100 μg/ml, 250 μg/ml

SELECTED DOSAGES: Divided daily dosing is recommended in infants and young children. The usual digitalizing and maintenance dosages for digoxin elixir and tablets for patients with normal renal function, based on lean body weight, are as follows. Consult manufacturer's information for IV and liquid-filled capsule dosages.

Age	Digitalizing Dose (μg/kg)	Oral Maintenance Dosage (μg/kg per day)
Preterm neonates	20–30	23–30% of oral loading dose
Term neonates	25–35	25–35% of oral loading dose
1–24 months	35–60	25–35% as above
2–5 years	30–40	Same as above
5–10 years	20–35	Same as above
>10 years	10–15	Same as above

COMMON SIDE EFFECTS: GI, CNS, visual disturbances with acute overdosage. Electrolyte disturbances with short- and long-term use.

SELECTED DRUG INTERACTIONS: Aluminum hydroxide, magnesium hydroxide, kaolin-pectin, magnesium trisilicate, and sulfasalazine reduce GI absorption.

CAUTIONS: Doses may require modification. Determine dosages with caution because digoxin has a low therapeutic index.

Dilantin: See **phenytoin sodium.**

Dilaudid: See **See hydromorphone.**

Diphenhydramine Hydrochloride

SYNONYM: Benadryl

CLASS: Antihistamine

DOSAGE FORM:
Capsules: 25 mg, 50 mg

Elixir: oral, 12.5 mg/5 ml

Injection: 50 mg/ml

SELECTED DOSAGES: Children >9.1 kg: 12.5–25 mg 3 or 4 times daily at 4- to 6-hour intervals. Children <9.1 kg: 6.25–12.5 mg 3 or 4 times daily at 4- to 6-hour intervals. Alternatively, for oral, IM, or IV therapy, children may be given 5 mg/kg daily or 150 mg/m^2 daily, divided in 3 or 4 doses.

COMMON SIDE EFFECTS: Children may have CNS stimulant effects or may be prone to more toxic effects than adults.

SELECTED DRUG INTERACTIONS: Additive sedative effects with other CNS depressant drugs.

CAUTIONS: Should be used with caution in infants and young children and should not be used in preterm or term neonates.

Diuril: See **chlorothiazide.**

Dobutamine Hydrochloride

SYNONYM: Dobutrex

CLASS: Sympathomimetic agent; adrenergic agent

DOSAGE FORM: Injection: 250 mg vial

SELECTED DOSAGES: Insufficient evidence to establish safety and efficacy in children. Neonates: 2–15 μg/kg per minute; titrate to desired response. Children: 2.5–15 μg/kg per minute; titrate to desired response.

COMMON SIDE EFFECTS: Ectopic heartbeats, increased heart rate, angina, chest pain, palpitations, increased blood pressure.

SELECTED DRUG INTERACTIONS: Effects may be antagonized by beta blockers such as propranolol and metoprolol.

CAUTIONS: Consult primary literature for use in children.

Dobutrex: See **dobutamine hydrochloride.**

Dopamine Hydrochloride

SYNONYM: Intropin

CLASS: Sympathomimetic agent

DOSAGE FORM: Injection: 40 mg/ml

SELECTED DOSAGES: Consult primary literature for dosages used in children. Neonates: 1–20 μg/kg per minute, continuous infusion; titrate to desired response. Children: 1–20 μg/kg per minute; maximum: 50 μg/kg per minute, continuous infusion; titrate to desired response.

COMMON SIDE EFFECTS: Ectopic heartbeats, tachycardia, angina, palpitation, hypotension, dyspnea, nausea, vomiting, headache.

SELECTED DRUG INTERACTIONS: Monoamine oxidase (MAO) inhibitors, alpha- and beta-adrenergic blocking agents, general anesthetics, phenytoin.

CAUTIONS: Insufficient experience to establish efficacy and safety in children by manufacturer.

Doxycycline

SYNONYM: Vibramycin

CLASS: Tetracycline

DOSAGE FORM:
Capsules: 50 mg, 100 mg

Injection: 100 mg

SELECTED DOSAGES: Consult references for specific infections. Usual dosage for children >8 years of age and >45 kg: 100 mg every 12 hours on first day, followed by 100 mg given in 1 or 2 divided doses; if <45 kg, then 4.4 mg/kg given in 2 divided doses on the first day, followed by 2.2 mg/kg daily, given in 1 or 2 divided doses.

COMMON SIDE EFFECTS: GI effects, nausea, vomiting, diarrhea, loose stools, anorexia, epigastric distress.

SELECTED DRUG INTERACTIONS: Antacids, oral anticoagulants.

CAUTIONS: Should not be used in children <8 years of age unless other drugs are ineffective. Retardation of skeletal development and bone growth in children could develop. Drug can cause tooth enamel hypoplasia and permanent yellow-gray to brown discoloration of the teeth.

Ecotrin: See aspirin.

Elavil: See amitriptyline hydrochloride.

Enalapril

SYNONYM: Vasotec

CLASS: Cardiac drug

DOSAGE FORM:
Tablets: (not scored) 2.5 mg; (scored) 5 mg; (not scored) 10 mg, 20 mg

Injection: Enalaprilat, 1.25 mg/ml

SELECTED DOSAGES: Safety and efficacy not established in children.

COMMON SIDE EFFECTS: Require discontinuance of drug in 3–6% of patients. Headache, dizziness, fatigue, hypotension, rash.

SELECTED DRUG INTERACTIONS: Lithium, diuretics, potassium-sparing diuretics.

CAUTIONS: Use with caution in renal impairment, sodium depletion, hypovolemia.

Endep: See amitriptyline hydrochloride.

Engerix-B: See hepatitis B vaccine.

Epinephrine

CLASS: Sympathomimetic-adrenergic agent

DOSAGE FORM:

Injection: 1/1000, 1/10,000

Inhalation: 2.25% racemic form (Vaponefrin)

Suspension: injection (as base suspended in 25% glycerin); ***not*** for IV use, 1:200 (Sus-Phrine)

SELECTED DOSAGES:

Severe Asthma or Anaphylaxis: Pediatric patients may receive 0.1 mg/kg (0.01 ml/kg of a 1:1000 injection) or 0.3 mg/m^2 (0.3 ml/m^2 of a 1:1000 injection) subcutaneously. Single pediatric doses should not exceed 0.5 mg. Doses may be repeated at 20-minute to 4-hour intervals, depending on the severity of the condition and the response of the patient. For prolonged effects, the 1:200 aqueous suspension may be given subcutaneously to children in single doses of 0.02–0.025 mg/kg (0.004–0.005 ml/kg) or 0.625 mg/m^2 (0.125 ml/m^2). Single doses as the aqueous suspension in children weighing ≤30 kg should not exceed 0.75 mg. Doses of the aqueous suspension in children may be repeated if necessary, but not more often than every 6 hours.

Severe Anaphylactic Shock: IV administration may be necessary because absorption may be impaired with subcutaneous or IM administration. If necessary, some clinicians recommend that children receive an initial IV epinephrine dose of 0.1 mg (10 ml of a commercially available 1:100,000 injection or of a 1:100,000 dilution prepared by diluting 0.1 ml of a commercially available 1:1000 injection with 10 ml of 0.9% sodium chloride injection), given over 5–10 minutes (the initial dose may have to be reduced in young children), followed by a continuous IV infusion at an initial rate of 0.1 μg/kg per minute; the infusion may be increased as necessary to a maximum of 1.5 μg/kg per minute. For advanced cardiac life support during cardiopulmonary resuscitation, epinephrine is preferably administered IV but may also be instilled directly into the tracheobronchial tree through an endotracheal tube or administered intracardially.

Cardiac Arrest: Usual pediatric IV dose: 0.01 mg/kg (0.01 ml/kg of a 1:10,000 injection). IV doses may be repeated every 5 minutes if needed. Pending further accumulation of data, the recommended pediatric dose for administration with an endotracheal tube is the same as for IV administration. Alternatively, the drug may be infused IV at an initial rate of 0.1 μg/kg per minute;

the rate of infusion may be increased in increments of 0.1 μg/kg per minute, if necessary, to a maximum of 1 μg/kg per minute. Pediatric intracardiac doses of 0.005–0.01 mg/kg (0.05–0.1 ml/kg of a 1:10,000 injection) have been recommended. The usual neonatal IV dose is 0.01–0.03 mg/kg (0.1–0.3 ml/kg of a 1:10,000 injection). IV doses may be repeated every 5 minutes, if necessary.

COMMON SIDE EFFECTS: Fear, anxiety, tenseness, restlessness, headache, tremor, dizziness, excitability.

SELECTED DRUG INTERACTIONS: Should not be administered concomitantly with other sympathomimetic agents because of additive effects and increased toxic effects. Should not be used in patients receiving other agents that can sensitize heart to arrhythmias.

CAUTIONS: Contraindicated in patients with shock (other than anaphylactic shock), organic heart disease, or cardiac dilation, as well as most patients with arrhythmias, organic brain damage, or cerebral arteriosclerosis.

Esidrex: See **hydrochlorothiazide.**

Feosol: See **ferrous sulfate.**

Ferrous Sulfate

SYNONYM: Feosol

CLASS: Iron preparation

DOSAGE FORM:

Liquid: concentrate, oral, 125 mg/ml (contains 27 mg elemental iron per milliliter)

Liquid: oral, 220 mg/5 ml (Feosol) (contains 47 mg elemental iron per 5 ml)

Liquid: oral, 300 mg/5 ml (contains 65 mg elemental iron per 5 ml)

Tablets: 300 mg (contains 65 mg elemental iron per tablet)

SELECTED DOSAGES: Children with iron deficiency should receive elemental iron in a dosage of 4–6 mg/kg daily, given in 3 divided doses.

COMMON SIDE EFFECTS: Constipation, diarrhea, dark stools, nausea, epigastric pain in 5–20% of patients. Ingest iron after meals, rather than between meals, to reduce side effects.

SELECTED DRUG INTERACTIONS: Tetracycline, chloramphenicol (avoid use in iron-deficiency anemia).

CAUTIONS: Large amounts of iron exert a strong corrosive action on the GI mucosa. Administration of iron preparations to premature infants, who normally have low serum concentrations of vitamin E, may cause increased red cell hemolysis and hemolytic anemia. Liquid iron preparations may temporarily stain dental enamel or the membrane covering the teeth of infants.

Flagyl: See metronidazole.

Fortaz: See ceftazidime.

Furadantin: See nitrofurantoin.

Furosemide

SYNONYM: Lasix

CLASS: Diuretic

DOSAGE FORM:
Injection: 10 mg/ml

Liquid: 10 mg/ml

Tablets: 20 mg

Tablets: (scored) 40 mg, 80 mg

SELECTED DOSAGES: Usually administered orally; may be given by IM or IV injection when a rapid onset of diuresis is desired or the patient is unable to take oral medication.

Edema: Infants and children: usual initial oral dose: 2 mg/kg as a single dose; dosage may be increased in increments of 1 or

2 mg/kg every 6–8 hours to maximum individual doses of 6 mg/kg. It is usually not necessary to exceed doses of 4 mg/kg or a frequency of once or twice daily.

Acute Pulmonary Edema Associated with Congestive Heart Failure: Infants and children: usual initial IV or IM dose: 1 mg/kg (use not included in FDA labeling). If necessary, for resistant forms of edema, the initial dose may be increased by 1 mg/kg no more often than every 2 hours until the desired effect has been obtained. Maximum individual doses for infants and children are 6 mg/kg; however, the potential risks associated with large parenteral doses of the drug should be considered and the patient should be monitored closely.

COMMON SIDE EFFECTS: Fluid and electrolyte depletion with large doses and in patients who have restricted sodium intake. Nausea, anorexia, oral and gastric irritation, vomiting, cramping, diarrhea, and constipation. Oral solutions contain sorbitol, which may cause diarrhea (especially in children) when high doses are administered. In children, mild to moderate abdominal pain has been reported after IV administration of furosemide.

SELECTED DRUG INTERACTIONS: Diuretics, drugs affected by or causing potassium depletion (cardiac glycosides), lithium, antidiabetic agents, hypotensives.

CAUTIONS: Watch for signs of hypovolemia, hyponatremia, hypokalemia, hypocalcemia, hypochloremia, and hypomagnesemia. Patients should be informed of the signs and symptoms of electrolyte imbalance and instructed to report to their physicians if weakness, dizziness, fatique, faintness, mental confusion, lassitude, muscle cramps, headache, paresthesias, thirst, anorexia, nausea, and/or vomiting occurs.

Garamycin: See gentamicin sulfate.

Gentamicin Sulfate

SYNONYM: Garamycin

CLASS: Aminoglycoside

DOSAGE FORM:
Injection: 10 mg/ml, 40 mg/ml: 60 mg, 80 mg syringe

Injection: for intrathecal use, 4 mg/2 ml

SELECTED DOSAGES: Gentamicin sulfate is administered by IM injection or IV infusion. For pediatric patients, the volume of infusion fluid depends on the patient's needs but should be sufficient to allow a gentamicin infusion period of 30 minutes to 2 hours. Children may receive 6–7.5 mg/kg daily, given in equally divided doses at 8-hour intervals; infants and neonates should receive 7.5 mg/kg daily, given in equally divided doses at 8-hour intervals; preterm or term neonates ≤1 week of age should be given 2.5 mg/kg every 12 hours. Peak and trough serum concentrations should be determined periodically, and dosage should be adjusted to maintain desired serum concentrations. In general, desirable peak serum concentrations of gentamicin are 4–10 μg/ml, and trough concentrations of the drug should not exceed 1–2 μg/ml. An increased risk of toxic effects may be associated with prolonged peak serum gentamicin concentrations >10–12 μg/ml or trough concentrations >2 μg/ml.

COMMON SIDE EFFECTS: Nausea and vomiting, anemia, leukopenia, granulocytopenia, thrombocytopenia; tachycardia and arthralgia less frequently.

SELECTED DRUG INTERACTIONS: Neurotoxic, ototoxic, or nephrotoxic drugs (other aminoglycosides, acyclovir, amphotericin B, bacitracin, capreomycin, cephalosporins, colistin, cisplatin, methoxyflurane, polymyxin B, and vancomycin should be avoided); neomycin, nonsteroidal anti-inflammatory agents.

CAUTIONS: Ototoxic and nephrotoxic effects are the most serious adverse effects. Aminoglycosides should be used with caution and in reduced dosage in preterm and term neonates <6 weeks of age because of the renal immaturity of these patients and resulting prolongation of serum half-life of the drugs.

Globulin, Immune Serum, Intravenous

SYNONYM: IVIG

CLASS: Serum

DOSAGE FORM: Injection: 0.5 g, 2.5 g, 5 g, 10 g, for IV use only

SELECTED DOSAGES: For primary immunodeficiency diseases: 100–400 mg/kg once monthly, depending on the particular manufacturer's product. For idiopathic thrombocytopenic purpura, 400 mg/kg daily, given for 2–5 consecutive days, depending on platelet count and clinical response.

COMMON SIDE EFFECTS: Adverse reactions seen in ≤10% of those receiving IVIG, and in <1% of patients without immunodeficiency. Most reactions are related to rate of administration rather than dose and may be decreased by reducing the rate of infusion or temporarily stopping therapy. Mild chest, hip, joint, back pain, myalgia, nausea, vomiting, chills, fever, malaise, fatigue, faintness, headache, flushing, and other effects have been reported.

SELECTED DRUG INTERACTIONS: Live virus vaccines should be administered at least 14 days before, or at least 6 weeks but preferably 3 months after, administration of immune globulins. Immune globulin may interfere with the immune response to certain live virus vaccines.

CAUTIONS: Contraindicated in people who have had anaphylactic or severe systemic reactions to immune globulin and in people with selective IgA deficiencies. The drug sometimes causes a precipitous fall in blood pressure. Observe closely the rate of infusion for each specific product because the products differ in dosage and infusion guidelines.

Glyceryl Trinitrate: See nitroglycerin.

Haldol: See haloperidol.

Haloperidol

SYNONYM: Haldol, Haldol Decanoate

CLASS: Tranquilizer

DOSAGE FORM:
Injection: 5 mg/ml, as decanoate 50 mg/ml

Liquid: concentrate, oral, 2 mg/ml

Tablet: (scored) 0.5 mg, 1 mg, 2 mg, 5 mg, 10 mg

SELECTED DOSAGES: Children 3–12 years of age and weighing 15–40 kg: usual initial oral dosage: 0.5 mg daily, given in 2 or 3 divided doses; subsequent dosage may be increased by 0.5 mg daily at 5- to 7-day intervals, depending on the patient's tolerance and therapeutic response.

Symptomatic Management of Psychotic Disorders: Children 3–12 years of age: usual oral dosage range: 0.05–0.15 mg/kg daily, given in 2 or 3 divided doses; however, severely disturbed psychotic children may require higher dosages. Dosage during prolonged maintenance therapy should be kept at the lowest possible effective level; once an adequate response has been achieved, dosage should be gradually reduced and subsequently adjusted according to the patient's therapeutic response and tolerance.

Nonpsychotic Behavioral Problems; Tourette's Syndrome: Children 3–12 years of age: usual oral dosage range: 0.05–0.075 mg/kg daily, given in 2 or 3 divided doses. Unlike psychotic disorders for which prolonged therapy is usually required, nonpsychotic or hyperactive behavioral problems in children may be acute; thus short-term administration of haloperidol may be adequate. The manufacturers state that there is little evidence that improvement in behavior is further enhanced at dosages >6 mg daily.

COMMON SIDE EFFECTS: Most frequent side effects involve the CNS. Extrapyramidal reactions occur frequently, especially during the first few days of therapy. They most often include marked drowsiness and lethargy, drooling or hypersalivation, and fixed stare; they are usually mild to moderate and reversible after therapy is stopped.

SELECTED DRUG INTERACTIONS: May be additive with, or may potentiate the actions of, other CNS depressants such as opiates or other analgesics, barbiturates or other sedatives, anesthetics, or alcohol. Lithium, anticoagulants, anticholinergic drugs, and methyldopa may also interact with haloperidol.

CAUTIONS: Shares toxic potential of phenothiazines. Safety and efficacy of IM administration of haloperidol lactate or decanoate injection in children have not been established, and those of other haloperidol preparations in children <3 years of age have not been established.

Heparin Sodium

CLASS: Anticoagulant

DOSAGE FORM:
Injection: 1000 units/ml, 5000 units/ml, 10,000 units/ml, 20,000 units/ml

Injection: for flush, 100 units/ml, 250 units/2.5 ml syringe

Injection: for flush, preservative free, 10 units/ml 100 units/ml

SELECTED DOSAGES: Full-dose continuous IV infusion therapy in children: some clinicians recommend an initial dose of 50 units/kg, followed by infusion of 100 units/kg given every 4 hours, or followed by 20,000 units/m^2 per 24 hours given by continuous IV infusion. Full-dose intermittent IV therapy in children: some recommend an initial dose of 100 units/kg, followed by 50–100 units/kg every 4 hours.

COMMON SIDE EFFECTS: Hemorrhage is the major adverse effect of heparin therapy. Bleeding complications occur in 1.5–20% of patients.

SELECTED DRUG INTERACTIONS: Drugs affecting platelet function (aspirin, nonsteroidal anti-inflammatory drugs [NSAIDs], dextran, dipyridamole), thrombolytic agents.

CAUTIONS: Avoid, whenever possible, heparin preserved in benzyl alcohol in the treatment of neonates. The use of heparin to maintain patency of umbilical-artery catheters reportedly has been associated with an increased risk of germinal matrix–intraventricular hemorrhage in low birth weight neonates; however, a causal relationship has not been definitely established. For severe hemorrhage, protamine sulfate should be given immediately.

Hepatitis B Vaccine

SYNONYM: Engerix-B

CLASS: Serum

DOSAGE FORM: Injection: 10 μg/0.5 ml vial, 20 μg/ml vial

SELECTED DOSAGES: Administer intramuscularly; ***do not*** inject intravenously or intradermally. It may be preferable to inject into the anterolateral thigh in neonates and infants, who have small deltoid muscles. Do not administer in the gluteal region; such injections may result in suboptimal response.

Neonates; Children ≤10 Years of Age: 10 μg at usual immunization regimen of 3 doses: first dose at elected date; second dose 1 month later; and third dose 6 months after first dose. Alternate schedule: Injections at birth and at 1 and 2 months of age are designed for certain populations (e.g., neonates born of hepatitis B virus–infected mothers, others who have been or might have been recently exposed to the virus, certain travelers to high-risk areas). On this alternate schedule, an additional dose at 12 months of age is recommended for infants born of infected mothers and for others for whom prolonged maintenance of protective titers is desired.

Children >10 Years of Age; Adults: 20 μg administered on either schedule.

COMMON SIDE EFFECTS: Local reactions at injection site, fever, headache, dizziness.

CAUTIONS: As with any percutaneous vaccine, epinephrine should be available for use in case of anaphylaxis or anaphylactoid reaction.

Hydralazine Hydrochloride

SYNONYM: Apresoline

CLASS: Hypotensive agent

DOSAGE FORM:

Capsules: 25 mg with hydrochlorothiazide 25 mg (Apresazide 25/25)

Capsules: 50 mg with hydrochlorothiazide 50 mg (Apresazide 50/50)

Capsules: 100 mg with hydrochlorothiazide 50 mg (Apresazide 100/50)

Capsules: 100 mg with hydrochlorothiazide 100 mg (Apresazide 100/100)

Injection: 20 mg/ml

Tablets: (not scored) 10 mg, 25 mg, 50 mg, 100 mg

SELECTED DOSAGES: Although the manufacturers have not established pediatric dosage recommendations, some clinicians recommend an initial oral dosage of hydralazine hydrochloride of 0.75 mg/kg daily or 25 mg/m^2 daily, given in 4 divided doses. An initial oral dose should not exceed 25 mg. If necessary, dosage may be increased gradually for a period of 3–4 weeks, up to 7.5 mg/kg daily. For parenteral therapy in children, some clinicians have suggested 1.7–3.5 mg/kg daily or 50–100 mg/m^2 daily, divided in 4–6 doses. An initial parenteral dose should not exceed 20 mg. If given with reserpine, the dosage of hydralazine may be reduced to 0.15 mg/kg or 4 mg/m^2 every 12–24 hours.

COMMON SIDE EFFECTS: Headache, palpitations, tachycardia, orthostatic hypotension.

SELECTED DRUG INTERACTIONS: Other diuretics, hypotensive agents, monoamine oxidase (MAO) inhibitors.

CAUTIONS: Patients with slow acetylation of hydralazine may have a higher risk of developing drug-induced systemic lupus erythematosus than patients with rapid acetylation.

Hydrochlorothiazide

SYNONYM: Esidrex, Hydro-Diuril, Oretic

CLASS: Diuretic

DOSAGE FORM:
Tablets: (scored) 25 mg, 50 mg

Tablets: (scored) 25 mg with reserpine 125 μg (Hydropres–25)

Tablets: (scored) 50 mg with reserpine 125 μg (Hydropres–50)

SELECTED DOSAGES: Children 6 months to 12 years: usual dose: 2–2.2 mg/kg or 60 mg/m^2 daily in 2 divided doses. Infants <6 months of age may require up to 3.3 mg/kg daily in 2 divided doses. Total daily dose may range from 37.5 to 100 mg for children 2–12 years of age and from 12.5 to 37.5 mg for children ≤ 2 years of age.

COMMON SIDE EFFECTS: Potassium depletion, anorexia, gastric irritation, nausea, vomiting, cramping, diarrhea, dizziness, vertigo.

SELECTED DRUG INTERACTIONS: Digitalis glycosides, corticosteroids, amphotericin B, lithium, antidiabetic agents, hypotensive agents, probenecid nonsteroidal anti-inflammatory drugs (NSAIDs).

CAUTIONS: Observe closely for electrolyte disturbances such as dryness of mouth, thirst, weakness, lethargy, drowsiness, restlessness, or oliguria—or muscle pains or cramps, muscular fatigue, hypotension, tachycardia, or GI disturbances such as nausea and vomiting.

Hydro-Diuril: See hydrochlorothiazide.

Hydromorphone

SYNONYM: Dilaudid

CLASS: Opiate agonist

DOSAGE FORM:

Injection: 2 mg/ml, 4 mg/ml, 10 mg/ml

Suppository: 3 mg

Tablets: 2 mg, 4 mg

CONTROLLED SUBSTANCE: Schedule II (C-II)

SELECTED DOSAGES: As an antitussive: usual oral dose in children >12 years of age: 1 mg every 3–4 hours. For control of cough, children 6–12 years of age have been given 0.5 mg orally every 3–4 hours.

COMMON SIDE EFFECTS: Dizziness, visual disturbances, mental clouding or depression, sedation, euphoria, coma, dysphoria, weakness, faintness, agitation, restlessness, nervousness, and seizures have been reported.

SELECTED DRUG INTERACTIONS: Other CNS depressants: opiate agonists, general anesthetics, tranquilizers, sedatives and hypnotics, alcohol, tricyclic antidepressants, monoamine oxidase (MAO) inhibitors.

CAUTIONS: Respiratory depression and circulatory depression are chief hazards of therapy.

Hydroxyzine

SYNONYM: Atarax, Vistaril

CLASS: Anxiolytic; sedative; hypnotic

DOSAGE FORM:
Capsules: as pamoate 25 mg, 50 mg (Vistaril)

Tablets: as hydrochloride 10 mg, 25 mg (Atarax)

Syrup: oral, 10 mg/5 ml (Atarax)

Injection: 25 mg/ml, 50 mg/ml (Vistaril)

SELECTED DOSAGES:

Symptomatic Management of Anxiety and Tension: In association with psychoneuroses and as an adjunct in patients with organic disease states who have associated anxiety: children ≥6 years of age: 50–100 mg daily given in divided doses; children <6 years of age: usual oral dosage: 50 mg daily, given in divided doses.

Pruritus Caused by Allergic Conditions: Children ≥6 years of age: 50–100 mg daily, given in divided doses. Children <6 years of age: usual oral dosage: 50 mg daily, given in divided doses.

As a Sedative Before and After General Anesthesia: Children: usual dose: 0.6 mg/kg orally or 1.1 mg/kg IM.

Nausea and Vomiting: Children: 1.1 mg/kg.

COMMON SIDE EFFECTS: Drowsiness, dry mouth.

SELECTED DRUG INTERACTIONS: Other CNS depressants: opiates, barbiturates, sedatives, anesthetics, alcohol; anticholinergic agents.

CAUTIONS: Drug may impair mental alertness or physical coordination. Use caution with IM administration because of adverse local effects (gangrene, thrombosis).

Hyperstat: See diazoxide.

Ibuprofen

SYNONYM: Motrin, Advil

CLASS: Analgesic and antipyretic

DOSAGE FORM:
Suspension: 100 mg/5 ml

Tablets: 200 mg, 400 mg, 600 mg, 800 mg

SELECTED DOSAGES:

Juvenile Rheumatoid Arthritis: Use is not included in labeling approved by the FDA. Children <20 kg: maximum dosage 400 mg daily. Children 20–30 kg: 600 mg daily. Children 30–40 kg: 800 mg daily. Children >40 kg have been given adult dosages.

Fever: Children 6 months to 12 years of age: usual oral dosage: 5 and 10 mg/kg for temperatures <39° and >39° C, respectively. Maximum daily dosage in febrile children: 40 mg/kg.

COMMON SIDE EFFECTS: Dyspepsia, heartburn, nausea, vomiting, anorexia, diarrhea, constipation, stomatitis, flatulence, bloating, epigastric pain, and abdominal pain. Most effects can be minimized by giving with meals or milk.

SELECTED DRUG INTERACTIONS: Anticoagulants and thrombolytic agents, other nonsteroidal anti-inflammatory agents.

CAUTIONS: Safety and efficacy in children <6 months of age not established. Should not be used as self-medication in children <12 years of age unless directed by a physician.

Imipramine Hydrochloride

SYNONYM: Tofranil

CLASS: Antidepressant

DOSAGE FORM:
Injection: 12.5 mg/ml

Tablets: 10 mg, 25 mg, 50 mg

SELECTED DOSAGES:

Functional Enuresis: Children at least 6 years of age: usual initial oral dosage: 25 mg daily, administered 1 hour before bedtime. If a satisfactory response is not obtained within 1 week, dosage may be increased to 50 mg nightly for children <12 years of age or to 75 mg nightly for children ≥12 years of age. Doses >75 mg daily do not improve results and may increase the risk of adverse reactions. For children who are early-night bedwetters, better results may be obtained by administering 25 mg in midafternoon and again at bedtime. Dosage for treating functional enuresis should not exceed 2.5 mg/kg daily. Once a satisfactory response has been achieved, the drug should be gradually withdrawn.

COMMON SIDE EFFECTS: Sedative and anticholinergic effects, postural hypotension, dry mucous membranes, blurred vision, constipation, urinary retention, drowsiness, weakness, lethargy, fatigue.

SELECTED DRUG INTERACTIONS: Monoamine oxidase (MAO) inhibitors, hypotensive agents, CNS depressants, antipsychotic agents, sympathomimetic and anticholinergic agents, cimetidine.

CAUTIONS: Although the clinical importance is not known, ECG changes have been reported in pediatric patients receiving twice the recommended maximum dosage. Safe use for the treatment of depression in children <12 years of age has not been established. Imipramine should not be used for the treatment of functional enuresis in children <6 years of age.

Imuran: See **azathioprine.**

Inderal: See **propranolol hydrochloride.**

Inocor: See **amrinone lactate.**

Intropin: See **dopamine hydrochloride.**

Isoproterenol Hydrochloride

SYNONYM: Isuprel

CLASS: Sympathomimetic

DOSAGE FORM: Injection: 1/5000

SELECTED DOSAGES:

Bronchospasm: Aerosol dose of *isoproterenol sulfate:* same for children as for adults, 80 or 160 μg (1 or 2 inhalations of a 0.2% suspension) by means of a metered inhaler; 2–5 minutes should elapse between the first and second inhalation. No more than 6 inhalations should be taken in any hour during a 24-hour period. Maintenance therapy: usually 80–160 μg (1–2 inhalations) 4–6 times daily.

COMMON SIDE EFFECTS: Nervousness, restlessness, insomnia, anxiety, tension, fear, excitement, palpitation.

SELECTED DRUG INTERACTIONS: Sympathomimetic agents, theophylline derivatives, general anesthetics.

CAUTIONS: Commercial formulations may contain sulfites, which can cause allergic-type reactions, including anaphylaxis.

Isoptin: See **verapamil.**

Isuprel: See **isoproterenol hydrochloride.**

IVIG: See **globulin, immune serum, intravenous.**

Kay Ciel: See **potassium chloride.**

Kayexalate: See **sodium polystyrene sulfonate.**

Keflex: See **cephalexin.**

Keflin: See cephalothin.

Labetalol Hydrochloride

SYNONYM: Normodyne, Trandate

CLASS: Hypotensive agent

DOSAGE FORM:
Injection: 5 mg/ml

Tablets: (scored) 100 mg, 200 mg, 300 mg

SELECTED DOSAGES: Safety and efficacy not established in children. Some clinicians have recommended initial oral doses of 4 mg/kg daily in 2 divided doses. Reported oral doses have started at 3 mg/kg daily and 20 mg/kg daily and have increased up to 40 mg/kg per day. IV intermittent bolus doses of 0.3–1 mg/kg per dose have been published. For pediatric hypertensive emergencies, initial continuous infusions of 0.4–1 mg/kg per hour with a maximum of 3 mg/kg per hour have been used. Use with caution because of limited data on its use in pediatrics.

COMMON SIDE EFFECTS: Dizziness, fatigue, nausea, vomiting, dyspepsia, paresthesias, nasal congestion, edema.

SELECTED DRUG INTERACTIONS: Halothane, cimetidine, glutethimide.

CAUTIONS: Safety and efficacy of labetalol, alone or in fixed combination with hydrochlorothiazide, not established in children.

Lanoxin: See digoxin.

Lasix: See furosemide.

Lidocaine

SYNONYM: Xylocaine

CLASS: Cardiac drug

DOSAGE FORM:
Injection: for IM injection 100 mg/ml

Injection: for direct IV injection 10 mg/ml, 20 mg/ml

Injection: for preparation of IV infusion: 2 mg/ml, 4 mg/ml, and 8 mg/ml in 5% dextrose

SELECTED DOSAGES: Controlled clinical studies to establish pediatric dosing schedules of lidocaine have not been performed. Some clinicians have suggested that infants and children may be given an initial IV bolus of 0.5–1 mg/kg; this dose may be repeated according to the response of the patient, but the total dose should not exceed 3–5 mg/kg. A maintenance IV infusion of 10–50 μg/kg per minute may be given with an infusion pump. For advanced cardiac life support in children, the recommended dosage is an initial IV bolus of 1 mg/kg. If ventricular tachycardia or ventricular fibrillation is not corrected after defibrillation (or cardioversion) and an initial lidocaine IV bolus, an IV infusion should be started at a rate of 20–50 μg/kg per minute; to ensure adequate plasma concentrations, an additional IV bolus of 1 mg/kg should be given at the start of the infusion.

COMMON SIDE EFFECTS: Serious adverse effects are uncommon and mainly involve the CNS. They include drowsiness, dizziness, disorientation, lightheadedness, and tremulousness.

SELECTED DRUG INTERACTIONS: Succinylcholine, antiarrhythmic agents, cimetidine, and propranolol may increase potential for a toxic reaction to lidocaine.

CAUTIONS: Safety and efficacy of lidocaine in the management of ventricular arrhythmias in children not established by controlled clinical studies. Use of the LidoPen Auto-Injector in children weighing <50 kg is not recommended.

Lithane: See lithium carbonate.

Lithium Carbonate

SYNONYM: Lithane, Lithobid, Lithocaps, Lithotabs

CLASS: Antimania agent

DOSAGE FORM:
Capsules: 300 mg

Liquid: lithium citrate 8 mEq equivalent to 300 mg lithium carbonate per 5 ml (Lithonate-S)

Tablets: slow release 300 mg (Lithobid Slow Release 450 mg; Eskalith CR)

SELECTED DOSAGES:

Acute Episodes: Although usual dosages of lithium salts for acute episodes in children have not been established, lithium carbonate dosages of 15–60 mg/kg (about 0.4–1.6 mEq/kg) or 0.5–1.5 g/m^2 (about 13.5–41.1 mEq/m^2) daily have been given in divided doses; however, the usual adult dosage should not be exceeded. When lithium salts are used in the treatment of children, dosage should be adjusted according to serum lithium concentrations, patient tolerance, and clinical response.

Maintenance Dosage: Although usual maintenance dosages of lithium salts in children have not been established, some clinicians recommend initial lithium carbonate dosages of 150–300 mg (about 4.1–8.12 mEq) daily, given in divided doses, and then dosage titration to achieve serum lithium concentrations of 0.5–1.2 mEq/L. Alternatively, lithium carbonate dosages of 15–60 mg/kg (about 0.4–1.6 mEq/kg) or 0.5–1.5 g/m^2 daily (about 13.5–41.1 mEq/m^2) daily have been given in divided doses; however, the usual adult dosage should not be exceeded. When lithium salts are used in the treatment of children, the dosage should be adjusted according to serum lithium concentrations, patient tolerance, and clinical response.

COMMON SIDE EFFECTS: Most often involve CNS, GI tract, and kidneys; are dose dependent; and generally occur at 12-hour steady-state serum lithium concentrations >1–1.3 mEq/L. Adverse CNS effects have occurred at serum concentrations <1 mEq/L, especially in children. Mild adverse CNS and neuromuscular effects initially occur in about 40–50% of patients. Lethargy, fatigue, muscle weakness, and tremor occur most frequently. As many as 40% of patients complain of headache, minor memory impairment and mental confusion, and/or a slightly decreased ability to concentrate. Hand tremor occurs in about 45–50% of patients and is usually benign. After 1 year of therapy, fewer than 10% exhibit tremor. Lithium has been reported to cause a variety of other adverse effects. Patients should be followed closely.

SELECTED DRUG INTERACTIONS: Thiazide diuretics: reduce lithium dose by 50% during treatment of lithium-induced polyuria.

Phenothiazines, nonsteroidal anti-inflammatory drugs (NSAIDs), and anticonvulsants have been known to interact.

CAUTIONS: Monitoring of serum lithium concentrations and of the clinical status of the patient is necessary in all patients receiving the drug. Instruct patients to avoid dehydration and to report polyuria and any prolonged vomiting, diarrhea, or fever.

Lithobid: See **lithium carbonate.**

Lithotabs: See **lithium carbonate.**

Loniten: See **minoxidil.**

Magnesium Hydroxide

SYNONYM: Milk of Magnesia

CLASS: Saline laxative

DOSAGE FORM:

Suspension: 77.5 mg/g

Concentrate: (10 ml is equivalent to 30 ml of regular)

Tablets: 300 mg, 600 mg

SELECTED DOSAGES: Laxative: children <2 years of age: 0.5 ml/kg/dose; children 2–5 years of age: 5–15 ml/day or in divided doses; children 6–12 years of age: 15–30 ml/day or in divided doses; adolescents ≥12 years of age: 30–60 ml/day or in divided doses. Antacid: children: 2.5–5 ml as needed.

COMMON SIDE EFFECTS: Laxative effect: frequent administration often cannot be tolerated; repeated doses cause diarrhea, which may cause fluid and electrolyte imbalances.

SELECTED DRUG INTERACTIONS: All antacids potentially may increase or decrease the rate and/or extent of absorption of concomitantly administered oral drugs by changing GI transit time or by binding or chelating the drug. Magnesium hydroxide (Milk of Magnesia) has the greatest potential for drug binding.

CAUTIONS: Monitor fluid and electrolyte balance.

Magnesium Sulfate

SYNONYM: $MgSO_4$

CLASS: Anticonvulsant

DOSAGE FORM: Injection: 10%, 12.5%, 50%

SELECTED DOSAGES: For IM use in infants and children, the drug concentration usually should not exceed 200 mg/ml (20%). Dosage must be carefully adjusted according to individual requirements and response, and administration of the drug should be discontinued as soon as the desired effect is obtained.

Acute Nephritis: In association with hypertension, encephalopathy, and seizures: children: 100 mg/kg (0.2 ml/kg of a 50% solution) has been administered IM at 4- to 6-hour intervals as needed. Children have also received magnesium sulfate IM in a dosage of 20–40 mg/kg (0.1–0.2 ml/kg of a 20% solution) as needed to control seizures. If symptoms are severe, the drug may be administered IV as a 1–3% solution in a dosage of 100–200 mg/kg. When administered by IV infusion, the drug should be given slowly and blood pressure should be closely monitored. The total IV dose should be administered within 1 hour, with half the dose administered in the first 15–20 minutes.

COMMON SIDE EFFECTS: Magnesium intoxication. Signs and symptoms of hypermagnesemia include flushing, sweating, hypotension, depression of reflexes, flaccid paralysis, hypothermia, circulatory collapse, depression of cardiac function, and CNS depression, which can proceed to fatal respiratory paralysis.

SELECTED DRUG INTERACTIONS: CNS depressants (barbiturates, opiates, general anesthetics, or other CNS depressants) will cause additive effects.

CAUTIONS: Administer magnesium salts with extreme caution in patients receiving digitalis, because serious changes in cardiac conduction with possible heart block may occur if administration of calcium is required to treat a toxic reaction to magnesium.

Mannitol

CLASS: Osmotic diuretic

DOSAGE FORM: Injection: 5%, 10%, 15%, 20%, 25%

SELECTED DOSAGES: Dosages for patients ≤12 years of age have not been established. However, some clinicians have suggested the following dosages for pediatric patients.

Oliguria or Anuria: Test dose: 0.2 g/kg or 6 g/m^2 given as a single dose over 3–5 minutes. Therapeutic dose: 2 g/kg or 60 g/m^2.

Edema or Ascites: Dose given as a 15% or 20% solution over 2–6 hours.

Cerebral or Ocular Edema: Dose given as a 15% or 20% solution over 30–60 minutes.

Intoxication: Drug given as a 5% or 10% solution as needed.

COMMON SIDE EFFECTS: Fluid and electrolyte imbalance. Acidosis, dryness of the mouth, thirst, urinary retention, headache, blurred vision, uricosuria, nausea, vomiting, rhinitis, arm pain.

SELECTED DRUG INTERACTIONS: Lithium excretion may be increased.

CAUTIONS: Mannitol should not be administered until the adequacy of the patient's renal function and urine flow has been established. A test dose may be used for this purpose. In patients with shock with oliguria and rising blood urea nitrogen level, mannitol should not be administered until fluids, plasma, blood, and electrolytes have been replaced. The cardiovascular status of the patient should be carefully evaluated before administration.

Medrol: See **methylprednisolone.**

Meperidine Hydrochloride

SYNONYM: Demerol

CLASS: Opiate agonist

DOSAGE FORM:
Injection: 50 mg/ml, 75 mg/ml, 100 mg/ml

Tablets: 50 mg

CONTROLLED SUBSTANCE: Schedule II (C-II)

SELECTED DOSAGES: Reduced dosage is indicated in poor-risk patients or very young patients. Children may receive 1.1–1.8 mg/kg orally, IM or subcutaneously every 3–4 hours as necessary. Alternatively, children may receive 175 mg/m^2 daily in 6 divided doses administered by the oral, IM, or subcutaneous route. Single pediatric doses should not exceed 100 mg. For preoperative doses, children may receive 1–2.2 mg/kg (maximum up to the adult dose) IM or subcutaneously 30–90 minutes before the beginning of anesthesia. As a supplement to anesthesia, meperidine may be given by repeated slow IV injections of a dilute solution (e.g., containing 10 mg/ml) or by continuous IV infusion of a more dilute solution (e.g., containing 1 mg/ml).

COMMON SIDE EFFECTS: Respiratory depression and, to a lesser degree, circulatory depression (including orthostatic hypotension) are the main hazards. Rapid IV administration increases the incidence of serious adverse effects. Dizziness, mental clouding, sedation, euphoria, dysphoria, nausea, vomiting, and constipation.

SELECTED DRUG INTERACTIONS: Other CNS depressants will cause additive sedative effects. The dose of meperidine should be reduced by 25–50% because these drugs potentiate the adverse effects of meperidine.

CAUTIONS: Observe patients closely for accumulation of normeperidine metabolites.

Mephyton: See phytonadione.

Methyldopa

SYNONYM: Aldomet

CLASS: Hypotensive agent

DOSAGE FORM:
Injection: 50 mg/ml

Suspension: oral, 250 mg/5 ml

Tablets: (film coated) 125 mg, 250 mg, 500 mg

Tablets: 250 mg with hydrochlorothiazide 15 mg (Aldoril-15)

Tablets: 250 mg with hydrochlorothiazide 25 mg (Aldoril-25)

SELECTED DOSAGES: In children, the usual oral dosage of methyldopa is 10 mg/kg daily or 300 mg/m^2 daily, given in 2–4 divided doses. Dosage is adjusted at intervals of 2 days until an adequate response is achieved. The maximum oral dosage for children is 65 mg/kg daily, 2 g/m^2 daily, or 3 g daily, whichever is least. The usual pediatric IV dosage of methyldopate hydrochloride is 20–40 mg/kg per 24 hours or 0.6–1.2 g/m^2 per 24 hours, administered in equally divided doses at 6-hour intervals. The maximum IV dosage for children is 65 mg/kg daily, 2 g/m^2 daily, or 3 g daily, whichever is least. When blood pressure is controlled, oral therapy should be substituted at the same dosage.

COMMON SIDE EFFECTS: Drowsiness that occurs in first 48–72 hours of therapy and may disappear with continued administration. Persistent decrease in mental acuity, including impaired ability to concentrate, lapses of memory, and difficulty in performing simple calculations, may occur and usually necessitates withdrawal of the drug. Nausea and nasal congestion are common.

SELECTED DRUG INTERACTIONS: Diuretics and other hypotensive agents may increase the effects of methyldopa. Phenothiazines and tricyclic antidepressants may decrease the hypotensive effects of methyldopa.

CAUTIONS: When methyldopa therapy is started, hemoglobin and hematocrit values should be obtained or a red blood cell count should be done and periodic blood cell counts should be performed during therapy to detect hemolytic anemia. Hepatic function should be checked during the first 6–12 weeks of therapy or whenever unexplained fever occurs.

Methylphenidate Hydrochloride

SYNONYM: Ritalin

CLASS: Cerebral stimulant

DOSAGE FORM:
Tablets: 5 mg, 10 mg

Tablets: sustained release, 20 mg

CONTROLLED SUBSTANCE: Schedule II (C-II)

SELECTED DOSAGES: Dosage must be carefully adjusted according to individual requirements and response. The extended-release tablet should not be used for initiating therapy nor until the daily dosage is titrated by using the conventional tablets; the extended-release tablets may be used and given at 8-hour intervals when the 8-hour dosage of the extended-release preparation corresponds to an 8-hour dosage of the conventional tablets.

Attention Deficit Disorder: As an adjunct in the treatment of attention deficit disorder in children ≥6 years of age, the usual initial dosage is 5 mg before breakfast and lunch. Dosage may be increased by 5–10 mg daily at weekly intervals. Some clinicians recommend an initial dosage of 0.25 mg/kg daily. If adverse effects are not observed, the daily dose may be doubled each week until the optimum dosage of 2 mg/kg daily is reached. Oral dosage in children should not exceed 60 mg daily. If a beneficial effect is not attained after appropriate dosage adjustment over a 1-month period, methylphenidate therapy should be discontinued. In children who have responded to methylphenidate therapy, use of the drug should be discontinued periodically to assess the patient's condition; improvement may be maintained temporarily or permanently after therapy is discontinued. Methylphenidate therapy should not be continued indefinitely and can usually be discontinued when the child reaches adolescence.

COMMON SIDE EFFECTS: Most adverse effects appear to be dose related and include nervousness and insomnia; they can usually be controlled by reducing the dosage and not administering the drug in the afternoon or evening. Other adverse effects include anorexia, nausea, abdominal pain, dryness of the throat, dizziness, palpitation, and headache.

SELECTED DRUG INTERACTIONS: Use cautiously in patients receiving pressor agents or monoamine oxidase (MAO) inhibitors.

CAUTIONS: Safety and efficacy of methylphenidate in children <6 years of age have not been established. Manufacturers recommend that laboratory tests, including periodic complete blood cell (with differential cell) and platelet counts, be performed periodically during prolonged therapy, although the clinical rationale for this regimen has been questioned. Refer to the literature for more information on this recommendation.

Methylprednisolone

SYNONYM: Medrol

CLASS: Adrenal hormone

DOSAGE FORM: Tablets: (scored) 4 mg, 16 mg

SELECTED DOSAGES: Methylprednisolone is administered orally. The route of administration and the dosage of methylprednisolone and its derivatives depend on the condition being treated and the response of the patient. IM or IV therapy is generally reserved for patients who are unable to take the drug orally or for use in emergency situations. After the initial emergency period, a longer-acting injectable corticosteroid preparation or oral administration of a corticosteroid should be considered. Some clinicians state that children may be given a dosage of 0.117–1.66 mg/kg daily or 3.3–50 mg/m^2 daily, administered in 3 or 4 divided doses. The dosage for infants and children should be based on the severity of the disease and the response of the patient rather than on strict adherence to dosage indicated by age, body weight, or body surface area. After a satisfactory response is obtained, dosage should be decreased in small decrements to the lowest level that maintains an adequate clinical response. When long-term oral therapy is necessary, an alternate-day dosage regimen should be considered. After long-term therapy, methylprednisolone should be withdrawn gradually.

COMMON SIDE EFFECTS: Short-term use, even in large doses, is unlikely to produce harmful effects. Long-term use, however, can produce a variety of devastating effects, including adrenocortical atrophy and generalized protein depletion.

SELECTED DRUG INTERACTIONS: Barbiturates, phenytoin, rifampin, estrogens, nonsteroidal anti-inflammatory drugs (NSAIDs), potassium-depleting drugs, vaccines and toxoids, oral anticoagulants.

CAUTIONS: Long-term use of pharmacologic doses in children should be avoided if possible because the drugs may retard bone growth. If prolonged therapy is necessary, the growth and development of infants and children should be closely monitored. High dosages in children may cause acute pancreatitis leading to pancreatic destruction. Children have had increases in intracranial pressure (pseudotumor cerebri), which have caused papilledema, oculomotor or abducens nerve paralysis, visual loss, and headache. Pseudotumor cerebri has occurred most frequently after reduction of dosage or a change in the steroid administered.

Patients should be continually monitored for signs indicating that dosage adjustment is necessary, such as remissions or exacerbations of the disease and stress (surgery, infection, trauma). Avoid commercial preparations of steroid-containing benzyl alcohol, which have been associated with toxic reactions in neonates after the use of large amounts (100–400 mg/kg daily) of benzyl alcohol.

Methylprednisolone Acetate

SYNONYM: Depo-Medrol

CLASS: Adrenal hormone

DOSAGE FORM: Injection: 40 mg/ml

SELECTED DOSAGES: Methylprednisolone acetate may be administered by IM, intra-articular, intralesional, or soft tissue injection. IM or IV therapy is generally reserved for patients who are unable to take the drug orally or for use in emergency situations. After the initial emergency period, use of a longer-acting injectable corticosteroid preparation or oral administration of a corticosteroid should be considered.

Systemic Effect: The IM dosage will vary with the condition being treated. When employed as a temporary substitute for oral therapy, a single injection during each 24-hour period of a dose of the suspension equal to the total daily oral dose is usually sufficient. When a prolonged effect is desired, the weekly dose may be calculated by multiplying the daily oral dose by 7 and given as a single intramuscular injection. Dosage must be individualized according to the severity of the disease and the response of the patient. For infants and children, the recommended dosage must be reduced, but dosage should be governed by the condition rather than by strict adherence to the ratio indicated by age or body weight.

COMMON SIDE EFFECTS: Short-term use, even in large doses, is unlikely to produce harmful effects. Long-term use, however, can produce a variety of devastating effects, including adrenocortical atrophy and generalized protein depletion.

SELECTED DRUG INTERACTIONS: Barbiturates, phenytoin, rifampin, estrogens, nonsteroidal anti-inflammatory drugs (NSAIDs), potassium-depleting drugs, vaccines and toxoids, oral anticoagulants.

CAUTIONS: The manufacturer of Depo-Medrol states that this formulation of methylprednisolone acetate should not be administered intrathecally because of reports of severe adverse events with such use. Long-term use of pharmacologic doses in children should be avoided if possible because the drugs may retard bone growth. If prolonged therapy is necessary, the growth and development of infants and children should be closely monitored. High dosages in the treatment of children may cause acute pancreatitis leading to pancreatic destruction. Children have had increases in intracranial pressure (pseudotumor cerebri), causing papilledema, oculomotor or abducens nerve paralysis, visual loss, and headache. Pseudotumor cerebri has occurred most frequently after reduction of dosage or a change in the steroid administered. Patients should be continually monitored for signs indicating that dosage adjustment is necessary, such as remissions or exacerbations of the disease and stress (surgery, infection, trauma). Avoid commercial preparations of steroid-containing benzyl alcohol, which have been associated with toxic effects in neonates resulting from use of large amounts (100–400 mg/kg daily) of benzyl alcohol.

Methylprednisolone Sodium Succinate

SYNONYM: Solu-Medrol

CLASS: Adrenal hormone

DOSAGE FORM: Injection: 40 mg/ml, 125 mg/2 ml, 1 g/16 ml

SELECTED DOSAGES:

Life-Threatening Shock: Some clinicians state that children may be given 0.03–0.2 mg/kg or 1–6.25 mg/m^2 IM 1–2 times daily.

Severe Lupus Nephritis: Although this condition is not listed in the approved FDA labeling, children have been given 30 mg/kg IV every other day for 6 doses. "Pulse" therapy has been followed by long-term oral prednisone or prednisolone therapy. The route of administration and the dosage of methylprednisolone and its derivatives depend on the condition being treated and the response of the patient. IM or IV therapy is generally reserved for patients who are unable to take the drug orally or for use in emergency situations. After the initial emergency period, a longer-acting injectable corticosteroid preparation or oral administration of a corticosteroid should be considered.

COMMON SIDE EFFECTS: Short-term use, even in large doses, is unlikely to produce harmful effects. Long-term use, however, can produce a variety of devastating effects, including adrenocortical atrophy and generalized protein depletion.

SELECTED DRUG INTERACTIONS: Barbiturates, phenytoin, rifampin, estrogens, nonsteroidal anti-inflammatory drugs (NSAIDs), potassium-depleting drugs, vaccines and toxoids, oral anticoagulants.

CAUTIONS: Long-term use of pharmacologic doses in children should be avoided if possible because the drugs may retard bone growth. If prolonged therapy is necessary, the growth and development of infants and children should be closely monitored. High dosages in the treatment of children may cause acute pancreatitis leading to pancreatic destruction. Children have had increases in intracranial pressure (pseudotumor cerebri), causing papilledema, oculomotor or abducens nerve paralysis, visual loss, and headache. Pseudotumor cerebri has occurred most frequently after reduction of dosage or a change in the steroid administered. Patients should be continually monitored for signs indicating that dosage adjustment is necessary, such as remissions or exacerbations of the disease and stress (surgery, infection, trauma). Avoid commercial preparations of steroid-containing benzyl alcohol, which have been associated with toxic effects in neonates resulting from use of large amounts (100–400 mg/kg daily) of benzyl alcohol.

MetroGel: See metronidazole.

Metronidazole

SYNONYM: Flagyl, MetroGel

CLASS: Miscellaneous anti-infective agent

DOSAGE FORM:
Injection: 500 mg

Tablets: 250 mg, 500 mg

Topical gel: 0.75%

SELECTED DOSAGES: The Centers for Disease Control and Prevention (CDC) recommends that children with trichomoniasis be treated with oral metronidazole.

Trichomoniasis: For the treatment of symptomatic and asymptomatic trichomoniasis: 15 mg/kg in 3 divided doses daily for 7–10 days. The CDC states that infants with symptomatic trichomoniasis or with urogenital trichomonal colonization beyond the fourth week of life can be treated with 10–30 mg/kg daily for 5–8 days.

Amebiasis: For the treatment of acute intestinal amebiasis, or amebic liver abscess in children, the usual dosage is 35–50 mg/kg given in 3 divided doses daily for 5–10 days. Some clinicians also recommend that children receive 1.3 g/m^2 given in 3 divided doses daily for 5–10 days. For the treatment of amebiasis caused by *Dientamoeba fragilis* (use not included in manufacturer's labeling), children have been given oral doses of 250 mg 3 times daily for 7 days. For the treatment of *Entamoeba polecki* infections in children (use not included in manufacturer's labeling), many clinicians recommend 35–50 mg/kg daily, given in 3 divided doses for 10 days, followed by oral diloxanide furoate, 20 mg/kg daily, given in 3 divided doses for 10 days.

Giardiasis: The CDC recommends that children receive 15 mg/kg in 3 divided doses daily for 5 days.

COMMON SIDE EFFECTS: With oral therapy, nausea often accompanied with headache, anorexia, dry mouth, and a sharp, unpleasant metallic taste.

SELECTED DRUG INTERACTIONS: Oral or IV metronidazole potentiates the effects of oral anticoagulants, resulting in prolongation of the prothrombin time; concurrent administration should be avoided if possible. Lithium serum levels may increase, resulting in a toxic reaction to lithium.

CAUTIONS: Manufacturers state that safe use of IV metronidazole in children for any indication and safe use of oral metronidazole in children for any indication except amebiasis have not been established; however, oral metronidazole has been used in children for indications other than amebiasis (e.g., trichomoniasis, giardiasis) without unusual adverse effects.

Minoxidil

SYNONYM: Loniten

CLASS: Hypotensive agent

DOSAGE FORM: Tablets: (scored) 2.5 mg, 10 mg

SELECTED DOSAGES:

Hypertension: Children >12 years of age: usual initial dosage: 5 mg once daily. Dosage may be gradually increased after at least 3-day intervals to 10 mg, 20 mg, and then 40 mg daily in 1–2 doses until optimum blood pressure response is attained. The usual effective dose in patients >12 years of age is 10–40 mg daily, and the maximum daily dosage is 100 mg. If rapid control of hypertension is required, dosage may be adjusted every 6 hours while blood pressure is monitored closely. Clinical experience for the management of hypertension in children, particularly infants, is limited and dosage must be carefully titrated. In children younger than 12 years of age, the usual initial dosage is 0.2 mg/kg (maximum 5 mg) once daily. If necessary, dosage is gradually increased after at least 3-day intervals in increments of 50–100% until optimal blood pressure response is attained. If rapid control of hypertension is required, dosage may be adjusted every 6 hours while blood pressure is monitored closely. The usual effective dose in children is 0.25–1 mg/kg daily in 1 or 2 doses, and the maximum dosage recommended by the manufacturers is 50 mg daily.

COMMON SIDE EFFECTS: Sodium and water retention occur frequently in patients receiving minoxidil and may result in edema, congestive heart failure, or pulmonary edema.

SELECTED DRUG INTERACTIONS: When administered with diuretics or other hypotensive drugs, the hypotensive effect of minoxidil is increased.

CAUTIONS: Clinical experience with minoxidil for the management of hypertension in children, particularly infants, is limited. In 3 pediatric patients who had received 40–50 mg of minoxidil daily for 47–158 weeks with other hypotensive agents, hypertensive encephalopathy occurred when minoxidil therapy was discontinued (dosage was decreased gradually over a period of 4–8 weeks); however, a causal relationship has not been established.

Moduretic: See **amiloride hydrochloride.**

Morphine Sulfate

CLASS: Opiate agonist

DOSAGE FORM:

Injection: 4 mg/0.5 ml, 4 mg/ml, 8 mg/ml, 10 mg/ml, 15 mg/ml, 25 mg/ml

Injection: preservative free, 5 mg/10 ml, 10 mg/10 ml (Duramorph)

Liquid: 20 mg/5 ml, morphine oral solution

Liquid: concentrate, oral, 20 mg/ml

Suppository: 5 mg, 10 mg, 20 mg

Tablets: 15 mg, 30 mg

Tablets: controlled release, 15 mg, 30 mg, 60 mg, 100 mg, MS-Contin

CONTROLLED SUBSTANCE: Schedule II (C-II)

SELECTED DOSAGES: Children may receive a subcutaneous or IM morphine sulfate dose of 0.1–0.2 mg/kg every 4 hours as necessary; single pediatric doses should not exceed 15 mg. IV doses of 0.05–0.1 mg/kg have been injected slowly in children, but this should be done carefully.

Severe, Chronic Pain Associated with Cancer: In a limited number of children, maintenance morphine sulfate dosages of 0.025–2.6 mg/kg per hour (median: 0.04–0.07 mg/kg per hour) have been infused IV, and dosages of 0.025–1.79 mg/kg per hour (median: 0.06 mg/kg per hour) have been infused subcutaneously.

Severe Pain Associated with Sickle Cell Crisis: Maintenance dosages of 0.03–0.15 mg/kg per hour have been infused IV in a limited number of children.

Postoperative Analgesia: Children have received maintenance dosages by IV infusion at a rate of 0.01–0.04 mg/kg per hour; however, because elimination of the drug may be slower in neonates and because neonates may be more susceptible to CNS effects of the drug, some clinicians suggest that the rate of IV infusion generally not exceed 0.015–0.02 mg/kg per hour in this age group.

COMMON SIDE EFFECTS: Respiratory depression and, to a lesser degree, circulatory depression (including orthostatic hypotension) are the chief side effects of opiate agonist therapy. Respiratory arrest, shock, and cardiac arrest have occurred. Rapid IV administration of opiate agonists increases the incidence of these serious adverse effects. Neonates should be observed closely for signs of respiratory depression if the mother has received opiate agonists during labor. Other adverse CNS effects include dizziness, sedation, visual disturbances, mental clouding or depression, coma, euphoria, dysphoria, weakness, faintness, agitation, restlessness, nervousness, seizures, and, rarely, delirium and insomnia. Adverse GI effects include nausea, vomiting, and constipation.

SELECTED DRUG INTERACTIONS: Potentiation of the effects of other CNS depressants, including other opiate agonists, general anesthetics, tranquilizers, sedatives and hypnotics, and alcohol, and of other CNS drugs such as monoamine oxidase (MAO) inhibitors, including procarbazine, has been seen. These drugs therefore should be used with caution and at a reduced dosage.

CAUTIONS: Safety and efficacy of morphine not established in neonates. Opiate agonists generally should not be used in premature neonates because the drugs reportedly cross the immature blood-brain barrier more readily than they do the mature barrier and thereby produce disproportionate respiratory depression. Opiate agonists should be administered with caution and in carefully determined dosages to infants and small children because these patients may be relatively more sensitive to opiates on a body-weight basis. Safety and efficacy of epidural or intrathecal injection of morphine in children have not been established.

Motrin: See **ibuprofen.**

MS-Contin: See **morphine sulfate.**

Mucomyst: See **acetylcysteine.**

Mucosol: See **acetylcysteine.**

Muromonab-CD3

SYNONYM: Orthoclone OKT3

CLASS: Unclassified therapeutic agent

DOSAGE FORM: Injection: 5 mg/5 ml

SELECTED DOSAGES: Safety and effectiveness not established in children. Although no adequate controlled studies have been conducted in children, patients as young as 2 years of age have received OKT3 with no significant adverse effects. Refer to clinical protocols. Some clinicians recommend IV doses in children <30 kg: 2.5 mg/day once daily for 10–14 days. Methylprednisolone sodium succinate, 1 mg/kg IV, given before the first muromonab-CD3 administration, and IV hydrocortisone sodium succinate, 50–100 mg, given 30 minutes after administration, are strongly recommended to decrease the incidence of reactions to the first dose.

COMMON SIDE EFFECTS: Pyrexia (90%), chills (59%), nausea (19%), vomiting (19%), chest pain, tremor, wheezing, headache, tachycardia, rigor, and hypertension, usually in the first 2 days.

SELECTED DRUG INTERACTIONS: Conventional concomitant immunosuppressive therapy should be lowered during OKT3 administration. Cyclosporine should be discontinued at the start of OKT3 therapy and resumed along with maintenance immunosuppression, if indicated, approximately 3 days before cessation of OKT3 therapy.

CAUTIONS: Only physicians experienced in immunosuppressive therapy and management of renal transplant patients should use OKT3. The drug should be administered in facilities equipped and staffed for cardiopulmonary resuscitation. In patients with fluid overload, severe pulmonary edema has developed during treatment with OKT3.

Mysoline: See **primidone.**

Nafcillin Sodium

SYNONYM: Unipen

CLASS: Penicillin

DOSAGE FORM:
Capsules: 250 mg

Injection: 500 mg, 1 g, 2 g

Tablets: 500 mg

SELECTED DOSAGES: The manufacturer of Unipen recommends an oral dosage of nafcillin for neonates of 30–40 mg/kg daily given in 3 or 4 equally divided doses. The usual oral dosage for the treatment of mild to moderate staphylococcal infections in children >1 month of age is 50 mg/kg daily, given in equally divided doses every 6 hours. Some clinicians recommend that children >1 month of age receive an oral dosage of 50–100 mg/kg daily, given in equally divided doses every 6 hours. The usual IM dosage for neonates is 20 mg/kg daily, given in 2 equally divided doses. Some clinicians suggest that when nafcillin is used IM in neonates, those <7 days of age receive 40–100 mg/kg daily in equally divided doses every 12 hours and those 7–28 days of age receive 60–200 mg/kg daily in equally divided doses every 8 hours. The usual IM dosage for children >1 month of age is 50 mg/kg daily, given in 2 equally divided doses. Some clinicians suggest that children >1 month of age receive an IM dosage of 50–100 mg/kg daily in equally divided doses every 6 hours for mild to moderate infections and 100–200 mg/kg daily in equally divided doses every 4–6 hours for severe infections. The manufacturers state that because of limited data on IV use of nafcillin in neonates and infants, IV dosage for these patients has not been established. However, some clinicians suggest that children >1 month of age receive an IV dosage of 50–100 mg/kg daily in equally divided doses every 6 hours for the treatment of mild to moderate infections and 100–200 mg/kg daily in equally divided doses every 4–6 hours for the treatment of severe infections, including osteomyelitis, pericarditis, or endocarditis, and that neonates receive an IV nafcillin dosage of 20.5 mg/kg every 8 hours. Alternatively, for the treatment of infections other than meningitis, some clinicians recommend that neonates ≤1 week of age receive 25 mg/kg every 8 hours (for those weighing ≤2 kg) or every 6 hours (for those weighing >2 kg), and that neonates >1 week of age receive this dose IV every 8 hours (for those weighing ≤2 kg) or every 6 hours (for those weighing >2 kg). For the treatment of meningitis, those neonates ≤1 week of age may receive 50 mg/kg IV every 12 or 8 hours, respectively, and those >1 week of age may receive this dose IV every 8 or 6 hours, respectively.

COMMON SIDE EFFECTS: Nafcillin shares risk with penicillins for hypersensitivity reactions, and therefore the usual precautions for penicillin therapy should be observed. Nausea, vomiting, epigastric distress, loose stools, diarrhea, flatulence.

SELECTED DRUG INTERACTIONS: Hypoprothrombinemic effect of warfarin may be decreased by nafcillin.

CAUTIONS: The manufacturers state that only limited data are available on IV administration of nafcillin to neonates or infants. If nafcillin is used in neonates, they should be monitored closely for clinical and laboratory evidence of toxic or adverse effects. In addition, serum concentrations of the drug should be determined frequently and appropriate reductions in dosage and frequency of administration made when indicated. Nafcillin that has been reconstituted for IM use with bacteriostatic water for injection containing benzyl alcohol should not be used in neonates because it has been associated with toxic effects. Renal, hepatic, and hematologic systems should be evaluated periodically during prolonged therapy.

Naloxone Hydrochloride

SYNONYM: Narcan

CLASS: Narcotic antagonist

DOSAGE FORM:
Injection: 400 μg/ml, 1 mg/ml

Injection: 20 μg/ml (Narcan Neonatal)

SELECTED DOSAGES: The commercially available naloxone hydrochloride injection containing 0.02 mg/ml is used for the treatment of asphyxia neonatorum; the 0.4 and 1 mg/ml injections are used in adult patients. However, because administration of unacceptable fluid volumes can result with use of neonatal naloxone hydrochloride injection (i.e., containing 0.02 mg/ml), especially in small neonates, the American Academy of Pediatrics recommends that use of this preparation be avoided when relatively large doses are used (e.g., those used in the treatment of opiate overdosage). When necessary, the more concentrated solutions also may be diluted with sterile water for injection to a concentration of 0.02 mg/ml.

Postoperative Opiate Depression: For partial reversal of opiate depression after the use of opiates during surgery, the usual initial dosage is 0.005–0.01 mg IV in children, given at 2- to 3-minute intervals until the desired response is obtained. Additional doses may be necessary at 1- to 2-hour intervals, depending on the response of the patient and the dosage and duration of action of the opiate administered.

Neonatal Opiate Depression: For reversal of opiate-induced asphyxia neonatorum, the usual initial dosage of naloxone hydrochloride is 0.01 mg/kg, administered into the umbilical vein of the neonate at 2- to 3-minute intervals until the desired response is obtained. Additional doses may be necessary at 1- to 2- hour intervals, depending on the response of the neonate and the dosage and duration of action of the opiate administered to the mother. When the IV route cannot be used, the drug may be administered by IM or subcutaneous injection.

Known or Suspected Opiate Overdosage: For the treatment of known opiate overdosage or as an aid in the diagnosis of suspected opiate overdosage, children may receive an initial IV dose of 0.01 mg/kg; if this dose does not produce the desired degree of response, a subsequent dose of 0.1 mg/kg may be administered. Alternatively, an initial 0.1 mg/kg IV dose, repeated as necessary, has been recommended for neonates and children up to 5 years of age, at which age a minimum 2 mg IV dose, repeated as necessary, can be used. When the IV route cannot be used in adults or children, the drug may be administered by IM or subcutaneous injection. Experience with continuous IV infusions of naloxone in children is limited, but children may require higher infusion rates (on a milligram-per-kilogram basis) than do adults. In several reports, infusion rates in children have ranged from 0.024 to 0.16 mg/kg per hour. Some clinicians recommend an initial pediatric infusion rate of 0.4 mg/hr.

COMMON SIDE EFFECTS: Tremor and hyperventilation associated with an abrupt return to consciousness have occurred in some patients receiving naloxone for opiate overdosage. Although no causal relationships have been established, hypotension, hypertension, ventricular tachycardia and fibrillation, and pulmonary edema have been reported occasionally in patients after postoperative administration of naloxone hydrochloride.

SELECTED DRUG INTERACTIONS: Use with caution in association with cardiotoxic drugs because serious adverse cardiovascular effects have occurred in postoperative patients after administration of naloxone.

CAUTIONS: When naloxone is used in the management of acute opiate overdosage, other resuscitative measures (e.g., maintenance of an adequate airway, artificial respiration, cardiac massage, vasopressor agents) should be readily available and used when necessary. Avoid excessive dosage after surgery; use with caution in patients with preexisting cardiovascular disease, and give with caution to patients known or suspected to be physically dependent on opiates (including neonates born to women who are opiate dependent), because the drug may precipitate severe withdrawal symptoms. Monitor patients closely because additional doses may be needed, the duration of some opiates possibly exceeding that of naloxone.

Narcan: See **naloxone hydrochloride.**

Nebcin: See **tobramycin.**

Neosar: See **cyclophosphamide.**

Netilmicin Sulfate

SYNONYM: Netromycin

CLASS: Aminoglycoside

DOSAGE FORM: Injection: 100 mg/ml, 1.5 ml vial

SELECTED DOSAGES: Netilmicin sulfate is administered by IM injection or IV infusion. Dosage is identical for IM or IV administration. Because netilimicin sulfate injections formulated specifically for pediatric use are no longer commercially available, particular care should be employed when one is preparing doses of the drug for neonates and young children with the 100 mg/ml injection. For IV infusions for pediatric patients the volume of infusion fluid depends on the patient's fluid requirements but should be sufficient to allow an infusion period of 30 minutes to 2 hours. For serious systemic infections (e.g., septicemia; skin and skin structure infections; intra-abdominal infections; lower respiratory tract infections), children 6 weeks to 12 years of age with normal renal function may receive 5.5–8 mg/kg daily, given in equally divided doses at 8- or 12-hour intervals. The manufacturer recommends that preterm and term neonates <6 weeks of age receive 4–6.5 mg/kg daily in equally divided doses at 12-hour intervals. Whenever possible, peak and trough serum concentrations should be determined periodically and dosage should be adjusted to maintain desired serum concentrations. In general, peak concentrations should be 6–12 μg/ml, with trough concentrations not to exceed 0.5–2 μg/ml. An increased risk of toxic effects may be associated with prolonged peak concentrations >16 μg/ml or trough concentrations >4 μg/ml. Consult appropriate references for dosing in renal impairment.

COMMON SIDE EFFECTS: Ototoxic and nephrotoxic effects are the most serious adverse effects of aminoglycoside therapy. Aminoglycosides also produce varying degrees of neuromuscular blockade. Some commercially available formulations of aminoglycosides contain sulfites, which may cause an allergic type of reaction in a small number of people, more frequently in individuals with asthma.

SELECTED DRUG INTERACTIONS: Additive neurotoxic, ototoxic, or nephrotoxic effects may be seen when netilmicin is given with drugs that have similar toxic potential (e.g., other aminoglycosides, acyclovir, amphotericin B, bacitracin, capreomycin, cephalosporins, colistin, cisplatin, methoxyflurane, polymyxin B, vancomycin), and they should be avoided, if possible. Aminoglycosides should also not be given with ethacrynic acid, furosemide, urea, or mannitol because of additive effects or altered serum and tissue concentrations of the antibiotics.

CAUTIONS: Like other aminoglycosides, netilmicin should be used with caution and in reduced dosage in preterm and term neonates <6 weeks of age because of the renal immaturity of these patients and the resulting prolongation of serum half-life of the drug. Each milliliter of netilmicin sulfate injection contains 10 mg of benzyl alcohol as a preservative. Administration of large amounts of benzyl alcohol (i.e., 100–400 mg/kg daily) has been associated with toxic effects in neonates and therefore should be avoided whenever possible. The American Academy of Pediatrics states that the presence of small amounts of the preservative in a commercially available injection should not prohibit its use when indicated in neonates.

Netromycin: See **netilmicin sulfate.**

Nifedipine

SYNONYM: Adalat, Procardia, Procardia XL

CLASS: Cardiac drug

DOSAGE FORM:
Capsules: 10 mg, 20 mg

Tablets: sustained release, 30 mg, 60 mg, 90 mg

SELECTED DOSAGES:

Hypertensive Emergencies: 0.25–0.5 mg/kg/dose.

Hypertrophic Cardiomyopathy: 0.6–0.9 mg/kg/24 h in 3–4 divided doses.

COMMON SIDE EFFECTS: Dizziness, lightheadedness, giddiness, flushing or heat sensation, and headache, reportedly occurring in up to 25% of patients, and, less frequently, hypotension (usually mild to moderate and well tolerated), weakness, peripheral edema, and palpitation. The incidence and severity of syncope, peripheral edema, and hypotension are generally dose related and occasionally may be obviated by a reduction in dosage.

SELECTED DRUG INTERACTIONS: Beta blockers, fentanyl, digoxin, H_2-receptor antagonists, anticonvulsant agents (phenytoin), hypotensive agents.

CAUTIONS: Blood pressure should be monitored carefully, especially during initiation of therapy and titration or upward adjustment of dosage.

Nipride: See **nitroprusside sodium.**

Nitrofurantoin

SYNONYM: Macrodantin, Furadantin

CLASS: Urinary anti-infective agent

DOSAGE FORM:
Capsules (macrocrystals): 25 mg, 50 mg, 100 mg

Suspension (microcrystals): 25 mg/5 ml

Tablets (microcrystals): 50 mg, 100 mg

SELECTED DOSAGES: Nitrofurantoin is administered orally and may be administered with food; the suspension is easily mixed with water, milk, fruit juice, or infant formula. Children and infants >1 month of age may receive 5–7 mg/kg daily in 4 divided doses. Therapy should be continued for at least 1 week and then for at least 3 days after sterility of the urine is attained. The manufacturers state that if long-term suppression therapy is used, dosage should be reduced. In children, dosage as low as 1 mg/kg daily, given as a single dose or in 2 divided doses, may be adequate. For long-term suppression therapy, some clinicians have recommended 1–2 mg/kg as a single evening dose.

COMMON SIDE EFFECTS: Nausea, vomiting, and anorexia. Side effects can be reduced by giving the drug with food or milk. The drug may turn the urine dark yellow or brown.

SELECTED DRUG INTERACTIONS: Uricosuric agents (probenecid, sulfinpyrazone), antacids, quinolones.

CAUTIONS: Nitrofurantoin is contraindicated in infants <1 month of age because of the possibility of hemolytic anemia as a result of an immature enzyme system.

Nitroprusside Sodium

SYNONYM: Nipride

CLASS: Hypotensive agent

DOSAGE FORM: Injection: 50 mg vial for dilution

SELECTED DOSAGES: A concentrated solution may be prepared by dissolving 50 mg of the drug in 2–3 ml of 5% dextrose injection. The manufacturers recommend that no other diluent be used. Other reports indicate, however, that sterile water for injection *without preservative* is suitable for initial reconstitution. Bacteriostatic water for injection should not be used for initial dilution because preservatives increase the rate of nitroprusside decomposition. *The concentrated solution should be further diluted in 250, 500, or 1000 ml of 5% dextrose injection to provide solutions containing*

200, 100, or 50 μg/ml, respectively. In adults and children not receiving other hypotensive agents, the average dosage of sodium nitroprusside is 3 μg/kg per minute, with a range of 0.5–10 μg/kg per minute; however, some patients will have profound hypotension when receiving the drug at this rate. Therefore the infusion should be ***started*** at 0.3 μg/kg per minute and gradually titrated upward every few minutes until adequate blood pressure control is achieved or the maximum rate of infusion of 10 μg/kg per minute has been reached. Diastolic blood pressure is usually decreased and maintained about 30–40% below pretreatment levels with sodium nitroprusside dosages of 3 μg/kg per minute.

COMMON SIDE EFFECTS: The first signs of overdosage with sodium nitroprusside are those related to severe hypotension. Increasing tolerance to the hypotensive effects of the drug and metabolic acidosis are also early indications of overdosage and may be associated with or followed by dyspnea, headache, vomiting, dizziness, ataxia, or loss of consciousness.

SELECTED DRUG INTERACTIONS: Ganglionic blocking agents, negative inotropic agents, general anesthetics (e.g., halothane, enflurane), most other circulatory depressants.

CAUTIONS: Profound hypotension and the accumulation of cyanogen (cyanide radical) are the most important adverse effects. Observe recommended maximum rates of administration. Frequent monitoring of acid-base balance is necessary in all patients because metabolic acidosis is one of the earliest and most reliable signs of cyanogen toxicity; however, acidosis may not occur until 1 hour after development of toxic cyanogen concentrations.

Normodyne: See **labetalol.**

Norpramin: See **desipramine.**

OKT3: See **muromonab-CD3.**

Omnipen: See **ampicillin.**

Oretic: See **hydrochlorothiazide.**

Oxacillin

SYNONYM: Prostaphlin

CLASS: Penicillin

DOSAGE FORM:
Capsules: 250 mg, 500 mg

Injection: 250 mg, 500 mg, 1 g, 2 g vials

Solution: 250 mg/5 ml

SELECTED DOSAGES:

Children Weighing ≥40 kg: Usual adult dosage of oxacillin for mild to moderate upper respiratory tract or skin and skin structure infections: 500 mg every 4–6 hours. When used orally as a follow-up to parenteral penicillinase-resistant penicillin therapy for the treatment of serious infections, give 1 g every 4–6 hours.

Children >1 Month of Age Who Weigh <40 kg: Usual oral dosage for mild to moderate upper respiratory tract infections or skin or skin structure infections: 50 mg/kg daily, given in equally divided doses every 6 hours. For follow-up of parenteral therapy for the treatment of serious infections, a minimum oral dosage of 100 mg/kg daily, given in equally divided doses every 4–6 hours, should be used. The usual IM or IV dosage for the same infections is 50 mg/kg daily, given in equally divided doses every 6 hours. For more severe infections, including lower respiratory tract or disseminated infections and osteomyelitis, the usual IM or IV dosage is 100–200 mg/kg daily in divided doses every 4–6 hours.

Neonates: IM or IV dosages of 25 mg/kg daily may provide adequate serum concentrations of the drug in some cases; however, some clinicians recommend that neonates ≤1 week of age receive IM or IV oxacillin dosages of 25–50 mg/kg every 12 hours (for those weighing ≤2 kg) or every 8 hours (for those weighing >2 kg), and that neonates >1 week of age receive 25–50 mg/kg IM or IV every 8 hours (for those weighing ≤2 kg) or every 6 hours (for those weighing >2 kg). The higher dosages are recommended for meningitis. Therapy should be continued for at least 1–2 weeks; more prolonged therapy is necessary for the treatment of osteomyelitis, endocarditis, or other metastatic infections.

COMMON SIDE EFFECTS: Adverse hepatic effects have been reported more frequently with IV oxacillin than with other commercially available penicillinase-resistant penicillins, including risk of hypersensitivity reactions. Other side effects include nausea, vomiting, epigastric distress, loose stools, diarrhea, and flatulence.

SELECTED DRUG INTERACTIONS: Rifampin, warfarin, probenecid.

CAUTIONS: Use usual precautions as for penicillin therapy. The manufacturers state that only limited data are available on the safety of oxacillin in neonates and that the drug should be used with caution in this age group. Transient hematuria, albuminuria, and azotemia have occurred in neonates and infants receiving high dosages of oxacillin (150–175 mg/kg daily). Elimination of penicillins is delayed in neonates because of immature mechanisms for renal excretion, and abnormally high serum concentrations of the drugs may occur in this age group. If oxacillin is used in neonates, they should be monitored closely for clinical and laboratory evidence of toxic or adverse effects, including renal impairment; organ systems (renal, hepatic, and hematologic) and serum concentrations of the drug should be monitored frequently and appropriate reductions in dosage and frequency of administration made when indicated.

Panmycin: See tetracycline.

Pemoline

SYNONYM: Cylert

CLASS: Respiratory and cerebral stimulant

DOSAGE FORM:
Tablets: 18.75 mg, 37.5 mg, 75 mg

Tablets, chewable: 37.5 mg

SELECTED DOSAGES:

Attention Deficit Disorder: To avoid insomnia and provide maximum effects during the waking hours, administer drug in the morning. Adjust dosage to individual requirements and response. Usual initial dosage for children ≥6 years of age is 37.5 mg daily, administered as a single dose each morning. The daily dose may be increased by 18.75 mg at weekly intervals until the desired clinical response is achieved. Effective doses usually range from 56.25 to 75 mg daily. Dosage in children should not exceed

112.5 mg daily. Beneficial effects may not be evident until the third or fourth week of therapy. In children who have responded to pemoline, the drug should be discontinued periodically to assess the patient's condition; improvement may be maintained temporarily or permanently after the drug is discontinued.

COMMON SIDE EFFECTS: Insomnia and anorexia, which appear to be dose related.

SELECTED DRUG INTERACTIONS: The interactions with other drugs have not been studied. Patients should be monitored carefully if pemoline is given with other drugs, especially drugs with CNS activity.

CAUTIONS: Safety and efficacy of pemoline in children <6 years of age not established. Prolonged administration of other CNS stimulants to children with attention deficit disorder has been reported to cause at least temporary suppression of normal weight and/or height patterns in some patients. Although a causal relationship between administration of CNS stimulants and growth suppression has not been definitely established, the possibility that growth may be suppressed during pemoline therapy should be considered, and patients receiving long-term therapy should be closely monitored. The manufacturer warns that pemoline may exacerbate symptoms of behavior disturbance and thought disorder in psychotic children.

Penicillin V Potassium

SYNONYM: Penicillin potassium, Pen-Vee K, phenoxymethyl penicillin

CLASS: Penicillin

DOSAGE FORM:

Solution: oral, 125 mg/5 ml, 250 mg/5 ml

Tablets: 125 mg, 250 mg, 500 mg

SELECTED DOSAGES:

Children ≥12 Years of Age: Usual adult dosage of penicillin V. For streptococcal and staphyloccal infections: 125–250 mg every 6–8 hours for 10 days, or 500 mg every 12 hours for 10 days. For mild to moderately severe respiratory tract infections caused by susceptible *Streptococcus pneumoniae:* 250–500 mg every 6 hours until the patient has been afebrile for at least 2 days. For mild skin and skin structure infections, 250–500 mg every 6–8 hours.

Children <12 Years of Age: Dosage should generally be based on weight. The usual daily dosage of penicillin V for the treatment of infections in children >1 month of age is 15–62.5 mg/kg (25,000–100,000 units/kg) daily, given in 3–6 divided doses; alternatively, a dosage of 0.5–1 g/m² daily, given in divided doses, has been used. For the treatment of group A beta-hemolytic streptococcal infections, the American Heart Association (AHA) currently recommends that children receive 125–250 mg every 6–8 hours for 10 days.

COMMON SIDE EFFECTS: Adverse local effects (phlebitis and thrombophlebitis) with parenteral administration, gastrointestinal (nausea, vomiting, epigastric distress, diarrhea) effects with oral administration.

SELECTED DRUG INTERACTIONS: Most drug interactions reported have involved penicillin G, not penicillin V, but the possibility that they may occur should be considered. Synergism with aminoglycosides, incompatibility with aminoglycosides, nonsteroidal anti-inflammatory agents.

CAUTIONS: Hypersensitivity reactions are one of the most frequent adverse reactions to penicillin G and penicillin V. Reactions vary from mild rash, eosinophilia, and fever to fatal anaphylaxis. Patients should be questioned in detail regarding a history of hypersensitivity to penicillins.

Pen-Vee K: See penicillin V potassium.

Pertofrane: See desipramine hydrochloride.

Phenobarbital

CLASS: Anticonvulsant; sedative and hypnotic

DOSAGE FORM:
Elixir: 20 mg/5 ml

Injection: 30 mg; 60 mg syringe; 65 mg/ml vial

Tablets: (scored) 15 mg, 30 mg, 60 mg, 100 mg

CONTROLLED SUBSTANCE: Schedule IV (C-IV)

SELECTED DOSAGES: Children: usual oral dosage: 3–5 mg/kg, or 125 mg/m^2 daily.

Febrile Seizures (Prevention): Maintenance dosage of 3–4 mg/kg daily has been effective. A period of 2–3 weeks of therapy may be required to achieve full anticonvulsant effects.

Status Epilepticus and Other Acute Seizure States: Children: phenobarbital sodium is administered parenterally in doses of 100–400 mg (20 mg/kg). Because up to 30 minutes may be required for maximum effect, it is important, in preventing overdosage, to allow the anticonvulsant effect to develop before administering additional doses.

COMMON SIDE EFFECTS: Drowsiness or sedation; however, in children the drug may produce paradoxic excitement and hyperactivity or may exacerbate existing hyperkinetic behavior, which is sometimes severe enough to necessitate a change to a different barbiturate derivative or another anticonvulsant.

SELECTED DRUG INTERACTIONS: CNS depressants, anticoagulants, corticosteroids, antidepressants, griseofulvin, doxycycline, anticonvulsants.

CAUTIONS: Phenobarbital shares the toxic potentials of the barbiturate-derivative anticonvulsants, and the usual precautions for anticonvulsant administration should be observed. IV phenobarbital may cause respiratory depression, particularly if administered too rapidly. Infuse at a rate no greater than 60 mg/min.

Phentolamine Mesylate

SYNONYM: Regitine

CLASS: Sympatholytic, adrenergic blocking agent; hypotensive agent; diagnostic agent for pheochromocytoma

DOSAGE FORM: Injection: 5 mg

SELECTED DOSAGES:

Pheochromocytoma (Diagnosis): Children: 1 mg IV or 3 mg IM. Alternatively, some clinicians have recommended an IV pediatric dose of 0.1 mg/kg or 3 mg/m^2.

Hypertension of Pheochromocytoma: For reduction of elevated blood pressure before surgical removal of a pheochromocytoma, children are given 1 mg, 0.1 mg/kg, or 3 mg/m^2 IM or IV 1–2 hours preoperatively; the dose may be repeated if necessary. During surgery for pheochromocytoma, 1 mg, 0.1 mg/kg, or 3 mg/m^2 may be given IV as needed to prevent or control paroxysms of hypertension, tachycardia, respiratory depression, convulsions, or other effects of excessive epinephrine secretion caused by manipulation of the tumor.

COMMON SIDE EFFECTS: Weakness, dizziness, flushing, orthostatic hypotension, nasal congestion, abdominal pain, nausea, vomiting, diarrhea.

CAUTIONS: Phentolamine may cause acute and prolonged hypotension, tachycardia, cardiac arrhythmias, and angina, especially after parenteral administration. If severe hypotension or other signs and symptoms of shock occur after administration of phentolamine, treatment must be vigorous and prompt and should include supportive measures; norepinephrine may be administered if necessary, but epinephrine should not be given.

Phenytoin Sodium

SYNONYM: Dilantin

CLASS: Anticonvulsant

DOSAGE FORM:

Capsules: 30 mg, 100 mg (in extended- or prompt-action formulations)

Injection: 100 mg/2 ml, 250 mg/5 ml

Suspension: oral, 30 mg/5 ml, 125 mg/5 ml

Tablets: (scored) chewable, 50 mg

SELECTED DOSAGES:

Seizure Disorders: Usual oral dose for children: 5 mg/kg or 250 mg/m^2 daily, administered in 2 or 3 equally divided doses. Total dosage should not exceed 300 mg daily. Subsequent dosage should be adjusted carefully and slowly according to the patient's requirements. Maintenance dosage for children usually ranges from 4 to 8 mg/kg daily. Therapeutic serum concentrations can be achieved more rapidly (in 2–24 hours) by using an oral loading-dose regimen. Various regimens have been suggested, and clinicians should refer to published protocols for more information. It is recommended that oral loading-dose regimens be reserved for patients in a clinic or hospital setting. In one regimen an initial oral loading dose of 500–600 mg (or 20 mg/kg) in children is administered in divided doses, followed by the usual maintenance dosage, beginning 24 hours after the loading dose.

Status Epilepticus: Children: usual dosage: 250 mg/m^2. Children may be given 10–15 mg/kg IV at a usual rate of 0.5–1.5 mg/kg per minute (maximum total dose: 20 mg/kg in 24 hours). Oral therapy should replace parenteral therapy as soon as possible.

COMMON SIDE EFFECTS: Nausea, vomiting, constipation, epigastric pain, dysphagia, loss of taste, anorexia and weight loss, mental confusion, nystagmus, ataxia, blurred vision, dizziness, insomnia.

SELECTED DRUG INTERACTIONS: Anticonvulsants, anticoagulants, antidepressants, chloramphenicol, antituberculosis, agents, doxycycline, amiodarone, digitoxin, CNS depressants.

CAUTIONS: Adverse effects are frequent and occasionally can be serious in nature, particularly when the drug is administered IV. If a rash appears during therapy, discontinue drug therapy. Most patients tolerate phenytoin blood concentrations <25 μg/ml. In some patients, serum levels >25 μg/ml are associated with nystagmus, ataxia, and diplopia. Serum levels >30 μg/ml are associated with drowsiness and lethargy, and rarely asterixis, may result; extreme lethargy and, occasionally, comatose states occur with >50 μg/ml.

Phytonadione

SYNONYM: Vitamin K_1, Mephyton

CLASS: Vitamin K

DOSAGE FORM:

Injection: 1 mg/0.5 ml, 10 mg/ml (AquaMEPHYTON)

Tablets: 5 mg

SELECTED DOSAGES: The minimum daily requirement of vitamin K has not been established but is estimated to be about 1–5 μg/kg for infants. The recommended daily dietary allowance (RDA) is 65–80 and 55–65 μg for males and females, respectively, ≥15 years of age; 5 μg for neonates ≤6 months of age; and 10 μg for infants 6–12 months. The RDA is 15, 20, 30, and 45 μg in children 1–3, 4–6, 7–10, and 11–14 years of age, respectively.

Hemorrhagic Disease of the Newborn: For prevention of hemorrhagic disease and for treatment of neonates whose mothers received anticonvulsant drugs during pregnancy, a dose of 0.5–1 mg should be given IM or subcutaneously to the neonate immediately after delivery and repeated, if necessary, 6–8 hours later. Rarely, it may be necesary to repeat the dose 4–7 days later.

Hypoprothrombinemia from Other Causes: For hypoprothrombinemia from malabsorption syndromes or from therapy with broad-spectrum antibiotics, salicylates, sulfonamides, quinine, or quinidine, infants may receive 2 mg and older children may be given 5–10 mg orally or parenterally. For patients receiving total parenteral nutrition, children may receive 2–5 mg IM once weekly.

COMMON SIDE EFFECTS: Severe reactions have occurred rarely during or immediately after IV administration; they have resembled hypersensitivity or anaphylaxis. Symptoms include cramp-like pains, convulsive movements, cardiac irregularities, chest pains, cyanosis, dulled consciousness, flushing of the face, dizziness, and rapid and weak pulse.

SELECTED DRUG INTERACTIONS: Because vitamin K_1 is a pharmacologic antagonist to coumarin and its derivatives, patients being treated with these anticoagulants should not receive phytonadione except for the treatment of excessive hypoprothrombinemia.

CAUTIONS: Hyperbilirubinemia and severe hemolytic anemia have been reported rarely in neonates, particularly in premature neonates, after large doses (10–20 mg). However, the incidence of these adverse effects is much less with phytonadione than with other vitamin K preparations. Each milliliter of AquaMEPHYTON contains 9 mg benzyl alcohol as a preservative. Toxic effects in neonates have been reported and appear to have resulted from administration of large amounts (i.e., 100–400 mg/kg daily) of benzyl alcohol.

Polycillin: See **ampicillin.**

Polymox: See **amoxicillin.**

Potassium Chloride

SYNONYM: Kay Ciel

CLASS: Replacement preparation

DOSAGE FORM:
Capsules: microencapsulated 10 mEq (Micro-K)

Injection: 2 mEq/ml

Liquid: oral, 15 mEq/11.25 ml, 20 mEq/15 ml, 30 mEq/22.5 ml, 40 mEq/30 ml

Tablets: for solution, 25 mEq potassium and chloride per tablet (K-Lyte/Cl)

Tablets: prolonged release, 10 mEq, 20 mEq (K-Tab; K-Dur)

SELECTED DOSAGES: Normal adult daily requirements and the usual dietary intake of potassium is 40–80 mEq; infants may require 2–3 mEq/kg or 40 mEq/m^2 daily. Potassium replacement requirements can be estimated only by initial clinical condition and response, ECG monitoring, and/or plasma potassium determinations.

COMMON SIDE EFFECTS: Nausea, vomiting, diarrhea, flatulence, abdominal pain or discomfort.

CAUTIONS: Administer with caution to patients with cardiac disease. Do not use in patients with severe renal impairment with oliguria, anuria, or azotemia.

Prednisone

SYNONYM: Deltasone

CLASS: Adrenal hormone

DOSAGE FORM: Tablets: (scored) 1 mg, 5 mg, 10 mg, 20 mg

SELECTED DOSAGES: Dosage depends on the condition being treated and the response of the patient. Dosage for infants and children should be based on the severity of the disease and the response of the patient, rather than on strict adherence to dosage indicated by age, body weight, or body surface area. Some clinicians state that children may be given a dosage of 0.14–2 mg/kg daily or 4–60 mg/m^2 daily, administered in 4 divided doses.

COMMON SIDE EFFECTS: Long-term administration of pharmacologic dosages of glucocorticoids to children should be avoided, if possible, because the drug may retard bone growth. If prolonged therapy is necessary, the growth and development of infants and children should be closely monitored. Alternate-day therapy minimizes growth suppression and should be instituted if growth suppression occurs. High dosages of glucocorticoids in children may cause acute pancreatitis leading to pancreatic destruction. Children have had increases in intracranial pressure, causing papilledema, oculomotor or abducens nerve paralysis, visual loss, and headache.

SELECTED DRUG INTERACTIONS: Hepatic microsomal enzyme inducers (barbiturates, phenytoin, rifampin) may increase glucocorticoid metabolism and therefore may require dosage adjustments if these drugs are added; nonsteroidal anti-inflammatory agents may increase the risk of GI ulceration; potassium-depleting drugs and other drugs that deplete potassium, such as amphotericin B, may enhance the potassium-wasting effect of glucocorticoids; vaccines and toxoids may have diminished response.

CAUTIONS: Short-term administration of glucocorticoids, even in massive doses, is unlikely to produce harmful effects. When the drugs are used for longer than brief periods, however, they can produce a variety of devastating effects, including adrenocortical atrophy and generalized protein depletion.

Primidone

SYNONYM: Mysoline

CLASS: Anticonvulsant

DOSAGE FORM:

Suspension: oral, 250 mg/5 ml

Tablets: (scored) 250 mg

SELECTED DOSAGES:

Children ≥8 Years of Age (and Adults): Usual dosage with no previous treatment: 100–125 mg at bedtime for the first 3 days, 100–125 mg twice daily for days 4–6, 100–125 mg 3 times daily for days 7–9, and then a maintenance dosage of 250 mg 3 times daily. Usual maintenance dosage: 250 mg 3 or 4 times daily. If necessary, dosage may be increased to a maximum of 2 g daily, given in divided doses.

Children <8 Years of Age: Usual dosage with no previous treatment: 50 mg at bedtime for the first 3 days, 50 mg twice daily for days 4–6, 100 mg twice daily for days 7–9, and then a maintenance dosage of 125–250 mg 3 times daily. Usual maintenance dosage: 125–250 mg 3 times daily or 10–25 mg/kg daily, given in divided doses. Alternatively, some clinicians recommend a dosage of 1.25 g/m^2 daily, given in 2–4 divided doses.

COMMON SIDE EFFECTS: Serious adverse reactions are rare, but mild adverse effects, such as drowsiness, ataxia, vertigo, lethargy, anorexia, and nausea and vomiting, occur frequently; ataxia and vertigo tend to disappear with continued therapy or with reduction of the initial dosage. Occasionally, primidone may cause hyperexcitability (especially in children), which may include hyperirritability; these effects are usually less severe than those seen with phenobarbital use.

SELECTED DRUG INTERACTIONS: Anticonvulsants, antidepressants.

CAUTIONS: Primidone shares the toxic potential of the barbiturate-derivative anticonvulsants, and the usual precautions for anticonvulsant therapy should be observed.

Procardia: See **nifedipine.**

Prochlorperazine

SYNONYM: Compazine

CLASS: Antiemetic

DOSAGE FORM:
Injection: 5 mg/ml

Suppository: 2.5 mg, 5 mg, 25 mg

Syrup: oral, 5 mg/5 ml

Tablets: (coated) 5 mg, 10 mg

SELECTED DOSAGES: Safety and efficacy in children <2 years of age or those weighing <9 kg not established.

Severe Nausea and Vomiting: Children >2 years of age and weighing >9 kg: usual oral or rectal dosage: 0.4 mg/kg or 10 mg/m^2 daily, given in 3 or 4 divided doses. Alternatively, the oral or rectal dosage in children >2 years of age and weighing 9.1–13.2 kg is 2.5 mg given once or twice daily but not exceeding 7.5 mg daily; children weighing 13.6–17.7 kg may receive 2.5 mg 2 or 3 times daily but no more than 10 mg daily; and children weighing 18.2–38.6 kg may receive 2.5 mg 3 times daily or 5 mg twice daily but no more than 15 mg daily. Generally, it is not necessary to continue oral or rectal therapy for longer than 24 hours in most pediatric patients. The usual IM dose in children ≥2 years of age and weighing >9 kg is 0.13 mg/kg. Generally, a single IM dose is sufficient to control nausea and vomiting in most patients.

COMMON SIDE EFFECTS: Adverse effects are numerous and may involve almost all organ systems. Extrapyramidal reactions, drowsiness, insomnia, restlessness, anxiety, euphoria, agitation, depression, weakness, dry mouth, blurred vision, hypotension (with parenteral administration), anorexia, constipation.

SELECTED DRUG INTERACTIONS: CNS depressants, anticonvulsants, lithium, metrizamide.

CAUTIONS: Phenothiazines should be used with caution in children with acute illnesses (e.g., chickenpox, CNS infections, measles, gastroenteritis) or dehydration, because the incidence of extrapyramidal symptoms, especially dystonic reactions and akathisia, is increased in these patients. Prochlorperazine shares the toxic potential of other phenothiazines. The incidence of extrapyramidal reactions appears to be relatively high in children. The drug's use should be avoided in children and adolescents with suspected Reye's syndrome because the antiemetic and potential extrapyramidal effects produced by the drug may obscure the diagnosis or be confused with the CNS signs of this condition; the drug also has hepatotoxic effects.

Propranolol Hydrochloride

SYNONYM: Inderal

CLASS: Cardiac drug

DOSAGE FORM:

Capsules: sustained release, 80 mg, 120 mg, 160 mg (Inderal LA)

Injection: 1 mg/ml

Liquid: oral, 4 mg/ml

Tablets: (scored) 10 mg, 20 mg, 40 mg, 60 mg, 80 mg, 90 mg

SELECTED DOSAGES: Although safety and efficacy have not been as extensively or systematically studied in children as in adults, current information from the medical literature allows fair estimates and specific dosing information has been reasonably studied. Weight-adjusted dosage in children serves as only an approximation for initial therapy, and dosage must be adjusted according to the therapeutic response of the patient.

Usual Pediatric Oral Dosage: 2–4 mg/kg daily, given in 2 equally divided doses as conventional tablets. Dosage should be calculated on the basis of weight rather than body surface area because the latter method may result in excessive plasma concentrations of the drug. Dosage must be individualized but should not exceed 16 mg/kg daily.

Hypertension: Children: oral therapy is usually initiated at 1 mg/kg daily, given in 2 equally divided doses as conventional tablets. Dosage should be titrated according to blood pressure response and patient tolerance. The antihypertensive maintenance dosage in children generally ranges from 1 to 5 mg/kg daily, given orally in 2–4 divided doses, although higher dosages occasionally may be necessary.

Supraventricular Tachyarrhythmia: Some clinicians state that pediatric oral dosages exceeding 4 mg/kg daily may be necessary for management. Oral therapy has been initiated at 1.5–2 mg/kg daily and titrated upward as necessary to control the arrhythmia, up to a maximum dosage of 16 mg/kg daily, given in 4 divided doses.

Tachyarrhythmia in Neonates with Thyrotoxicosis: An oral dosage of 2 mg/kg daily, given in 2–4 divided doses, has been used, although higher dosages occasionally may be needed (not included currently in FDA labeling). Although parenteral therapy currently is not recommended by the manufacturer for use in children, an initial IV dose of 10–20 μg/kg infused over 10 minutes has been recommended by some clinicians. Dilutions should be based on the 1 mg/ml dosage form (1000 μg/ml or 100 μg/0.1 ml).

COMMON SIDE EFFECTS: Bradycardia, hypotension, syncope, lightheadedness, giddiness, ataxia, dizziness, irritability, sleepiness, weakness, fatigue.

SELECTED DRUG INTERACTIONS: Phenothiazines, antipsychotic agents, sympathomimetic agents, antimuscarinic agents and drugs with anticholinergic effects, diuretics and cardiovascular drugs, neuromuscular blocking agents, ergot alkaloids, cimetidine.

CAUTIONS: Adverse reactions are more frequent and may be more severe after IV administration. Use with care in patients with inadequate cardiac function. ***Avoid abrupt withdrawal of the drug.*** Cardiovascular diseases that are common to adults and children generally are as responsive to propranolol therapy in children as in adults, and adverse reactions also are similar. Effects in Down's syndrome may be more pronounced. Safety and efficacy of extended-release capsules, oral solution, and injection have not been established in children.

Prostaphlin: See **oxacillin.**

Proventil: See **albuterol.**

Regitine: See **phentolamine mesylate.**

Rifadin: See **rifampin.**

Rifampin

SYNONYM: Rifadin, Rimactane

CLASS: Antitubercular agent

DOSAGE FORM:
Capsules: 300 mg

Injection: 600 mg/vial

SELECTED DOSAGES: Rifampin is usually administered orally. When oral therapy is not feasible, the drug may be given by IV infusion. Rifampin should ***not*** be given IM or subcutaneously. Oral therapy should be given 1 hour before or 2 hours after ingestion of food to ensure maximum absorption. For IV infusion, rifampin powder for injection should be reconstituted by adding 10 ml of sterile water for injection to the vial labeled as containing 600 mg to provide a solution containing 60 mg/ml. The appropriate dose of reconstituted solution may then be added to 500 ml of 5% dextrose injection and infused at a rate that allows complete infusion within 3 hours. Alternatively, the dose of reconstituted solution may be added to 100 ml of 5% dextrose injection and infused at a rate that allows complete infusion within 30 minutes.

Tuberculosis: Children may be given 10–20 mg/kg daily; dosage should not exceed 600 mg daily. Some clinicians recommend a maximum dosage of 10 mg/kg daily in neonates <1 week of age. When rifampin is used in combination with isoniazid in children, limiting rifampin dosage to 15 mg/kg daily and isoniazid dosage to 10 mg/kg daily may minimize the risk of hepatotoxic effects. If short-course therapy is used in children, rifampin and isoniazid dosages of 10–15 mg/kg (up to 600 mg) daily and 10 mg/kg (up to 300 mg) daily, respectively, are suggested. A short-course regimen consisting of daily administration of 10–20 mg/kg of rifampin (up to 600 mg) and 10–20 mg/kg of isoniazid (up to 300 mg) for 1–2 months, followed by twice-weekly administration of 10–20 mg/kg of rifampin (up to 600 mg) and 20–40 mg/kg of isoniazid (up to 900 mg) to complete a 9-month treatment period, may also be used in children. If an additional anti-infective agent is necessary initially for possibly resistant *Mycobacterium tuberculosis*, ethambutol, 15–25 mg/kg (up to 2.5 g) daily, may be used in children whose visual acuity can be monitored; in children whose visual acuity cannot be monitored carefully (e.g., very young children), pyrazinamide, 15–30 mg/kg (up to 2 g) daily, or IM streptomycin, 20–40 mg/kg (up to 1 g) daily, may be given until initial drug susceptibility to rifampin and isoniazid is confirmed. Short-course therapy with rifampin and isoniazid generally has been continued for a minimum of 9 months in children; however, 6-month regimens probably are as effective in children as in adults.

Asymptomatic Meningococcus (Carriers): When rifampin is

used to eliminate meningococci from the nasopharynx of symptom-free *Neisseria meningitidis* carriers, the American Academy of Pediatrics and the manufacturer of Rifadin recommended that children ≥1 month of age receive 10 mg/kg twice daily for 2 days and that children <1 month of age receive 5 mg/kg twice daily for 2 days. Alternatively, the manufacturer of Rimactane recommends that children receive 10–20 mg/kg once daily (up to 600 mg) for 4 days.

***Haemophilus Influenzae* Type b infection (Prophylaxis):** Children: recommended dosage: 20 mg/kg (up to 600 mg) once daily for 4 consecutive days. Dosage for very young infants has not been established, but some clinicians recommend a dosage of 10 mg/kg once daily for 4 consecutive days in neonates (≤1 month of age).

COMMON SIDE EFFECTS: Heartburn, epigastric distress, nausea, anorexia, abdominal cramps, flatulence, diarrhea. These effects can be minimized by administering the drug during or immediately after a meal. Headache, drowsiness, fatigue, ataxia, dizziness, mental confusion, visual disturbances.

SELECTED DRUG INTERACTIONS: Aminosalicylic acid, barbiturates, diazepam, clofibrate, disopyramide, mexiletine, theophylline, verapamil, clofazimine, ketoconazole, probenecid.

CAUTIONS: Rifampin and its metabolites may result in red-orange urine, feces, sputum, sweat, and tears; patients should be informed of this possibility. Soft contact lenses may become permanently stained.

Rimactane: See **rifampin.**

Ritalin: See **methylphenidate hydrochloride.**

Rocephin: See **ceftriaxone.**

Septra: See **trimethoprim-sulfamethoxazole.**

Sodium Polystyrene Sulfonate

SYNONYM: Kayexalate

CLASS: Potassium-removing resin

DOSAGE FORM: Liquid: oral, 25%; each 60 ml contains 15 g and 14.1 g sorbitol

SELECTED DOSAGES: Dosage must be individualized because it depends on the daily assessment of total body potassium. Pediatric dosage may be based on the fact that 1 g of the resin binds approximately 1 mEq of potassium. When given orally, each dose of the powdered resin is usually given as a suspension in water or in a syrup such as 70% sorbitol; usually 20–100 ml of fluid is used.

COMMON SIDE EFFECTS: Gastric irritation, anorexia, nausea, vomiting, constipation.

SELECTED DRUG INTERACTIONS: Magnesium hydroxide and calcium carbonate have been reported to cause metabolic alkalosis in patients with renal disease.

CAUTIONS: Large oral doses may cause fecal impaction. Patients should be monitored for electrolyte abnormalities.

Solu-Medrol: See **methylprednisolone sodium succinate.**

Somophyllin: See **aminophylline.**

Sumycin: See **tetracycline.**

Suprax: See **cefixime.**

Symmetrel: See **amantadine hydrochloride.**

Tazicef: See **ceftazidime.**

Tazidime: See **ceftazidime.**

Tegretol: See **carbamazepine.**

Tempra: See **acetaminophen.**

Tenormin: See **atenolol.**

Tetracycline

SYNONYM: Achromycin, Panmycin, Sumycin

CLASS: Tetracycline

DOSAGE FORM:
Capsules: 250 mg, 500 mg

Injection: for IM use only: 100 mg, 250 mg

Injection: for IV use only: 500 mg

Suspension: oral, 125 mg/5 ml

SELECTED DOSAGES:

Children >8 Years of Age: Usual oral dosage: 25–50 mg/kg daily given in 2–4 divided doses. Alternatively, some clinicians recommend that children receive 0.6–1.2 g/m^2 daily. The usual IV dosage is 12 mg/kg daily, given in 2 divided doses, but 10–20 mg/kg may be given daily depending on the severity of the infection. The usual IM dosage is 15–25 mg/kg daily, given in 2 or 3 divided doses with a maximum dosage of 250 mg as a single daily injection.

COMMON SIDE EFFECTS: Dose-related GI effects, including nausea, vomiting, diarrhea, bulky loose stools, anorexia, flatulence, abdominal discomfort, epigastric burning and distress, photosensitivity.

SELECTED DRUG INTERACTIONS: Cations (antacids containing aluminum, calcium, or magnesium), drugs affecting GI pH, oral anticoagulants, kaolin, pectin, barbiturates, phenytoin, carbamazepine, lithium.

CAUTIONS: Tetracyclines should not be used in women during pregnancy or in children <9 years of age unless other appropriate drugs are ineffective or are contraindicated. The American Academy of Pediatrics recommends that tetracyclines be used only in children who are ≥9 years of age, except under unusual circumstances. Their use could result in retardation of skeletal development and bone growth in the fetus or child, or in hypoplasia and permanent yellow-gray to brown discoloration of the teeth if used during pregnancy or in children ≤4–6 months of age.

Theo-Dur: See **theophylline.**

Theolair: See **theophylline.**

Theophylline

SYNONYM: Theolair, Theo-Dur, Uniphyl

CLASS: Respiratory smooth muscle relaxant

DOSAGE FORM:

Parenteral injection for IV infusion: 400 mg and 800 mg in various concentrations in 5% dextrose

Liquid: alcohol-free solution, 80 mg/15 ml

Tablets: (scored) Rapid Release, 125 mg, 250 mg (Theolair)

Tablets: (scored) Prolonged Action, 100 mg, 200 mg, 300 mg (Theo-Dur); 400 mg (Uniphyl)

SELECTED DOSAGES:

Acute Bronchospasm: For the treatment of acute bronchospasm, theophylline (often as aminophylline) is preferably administered IV. Only the injection containing approximately 20 mg of theophylline (25 mg of aminophylline) per milliliter should be administered IV. To minimize adverse effects, one should administer IV theophylline slowly, at a rate not exceeding 20 mg/min; loading doses are usually given over 20–30 minutes. If patients have acute adverse effects while loading doses of theophylline are being infused, the infusion may be stopped for 5–10 minutes or administered at a slower rate.

Patients not currently receiving theophylline preparations may receive a theophylline loading dose of 4.7 mg/kg (approximately equivalent to hydrous aminophylline, 6 mg/kg) and the following maintenance dosages IV:

Approximate IV Theophylline Dosage for Treatment of Acute Bronchospasm

Group	Maintenance Dosage for Next 12 Hours	Maintenance Dosage after 12 Hours
Children 6 months to 9 years of age	0.95 mg/kg per hour (1.2 mg/kg per hour)*	0.79 mg/kg per hour (1 mg/kg per hour)*
Children 9–16 years of age and young adult smokers	0.79 mg/kg per hour (1 mg/kg per hour)*	0.63 mg/kg per hour (0.8 mg/kg per hour)*

*Equivalent hydrous aminophylline dosage indicated in parentheses.

In *patients who are currently receiving theophylline preparations,* the time, amount, route of administration, and dosage form of the patient's last dose should be determined when possible and considered in determining a loading dose. Loading doses are based on the general expectation that each 0.5 mg of theophylline per kilogram of lean body weight will result in a 1 μg/ml increase in serum theophylline concentration. Ideally, in patients who are currently receiving theophylline preparations, the loading dose should be deferred until a serum theophylline concentration can be attained rapidly; when this is not possible, the clinician must carefully select a dose based on the potential benefits and risks. When there is sufficient respiratory distress in these patients to warrant a small risk, a theophylline loading dose of 2.5 mg/kg may be administered; this dose is likely to increase serum concentrations by about 5 μg/ml and is unlikely to result in dangerous adverse effects if the patient does not currently have theophylline toxic effects. Maintenance dosage should be decreased if adverse effects occur.

Because of the marked variation in theophylline metabolism in children <6 months of age, the manufacturers recommend that theophylline not be administered to these children. However, it has been used in this age group, and specialized references should be consulted for dosage information.

Although IV theophylline is preferred for the treatment of acute bronchospasm, oral solutions or suspensions of the drug or plain, uncoated tablets may also be administered. Other oral dosage forms (e.g., extended-release preparations) should ***not*** be used for acute bronchospasm. *Patients not currently receiving theophylline preparations* may receive a theophylline loading dose of 6 mg/kg and the following maintenance dosages orally:

Approximate Oral Theophylline Dosage for Treatment of Acute Bronchospasm

Group	Dosage for Next 12–16 Hours	Maintenance Dosage
Children 6 months to 9 years of age	4 mg/kg every 4 hours × 3 doses	4 mg/kg every 6 hours
Children 9–16 years of age and young adult smokers	3 mg/kg every 4 hours × 3 doses	3 mg/kg every 6 hours

In *patients who are currently receiving theophylline preparations*, a modified loading dose (same as with parenteral therapy) may be administered if warranted; maintenance dosages in these patients are the same as those for patients not currently receiving theophylline preparations and should be decreased if adverse effects occur.

Chronic Bronchospasm: Rapidly absorbed dosage forms: usual initial oral dosage of theophylline: 16 mg/kg or 400 mg daily (whichever is less), given in 3 or 4 divided doses at 6- to 8-hour intervals. Although extended-release preparations have been formulated to release the drug at various rates suitable for dosing every 8–12, 12, or 24 hours, the actual dosing frequency for a given patient and preparation depends on the patient's individual pharmacokinetic parameters. When extended-release preparations are administered, the usual initial oral dosage of theophylline in children and adults is 12 mg/kg or 400 mg daily (whichever is less), given in 2 or 3 divided doses at 8- or 12-hour intervals. With rapidly absorbed dosage forms, the dosage may be increased, if tolerated, in approximate increments of 25% at 2- to 3-day intervals. With extended-release preparations, dosage may be increased, if tolerated, by 2–3 mg/kg daily at 3-day intervals.

Regardless of dosage form, dosage may be increased, if tolerated, up to the following maximum daily doses, without measurement of serum theophylline concentration:

Children <9 years of age	24 mg/kg daily
Children 9–12 years of age	20 mg/kg daily
Patients 12–16 years of age	18 mg/kg daily
Patients ≥16 years of age	13 mg/kg or 900 mg daily (whichever is less)

Dosage adjustments may be based on peak serum theophylline concentrations and the clinical response and tolerance of the patient, as follows:

Dosage Adjustment After Serum Theophylline Measurement

If Serum Level of Theophylline Is	Serum Level	Directions
Within normal limits	10–20 μg/ml	Maintain dosage if tolerated; recheck serum theophylline concentration at 6- to 12-month intervals*
Too high	20–25 μg/ml	Decrease doses by about 10%; recheck serum theophylline concentration after 3 days and then at 6- to 12-month intervals*
	25–30 μg/ml	Skip next dose and decrease subsequent doses by 25%; recheck serum theophylline level
	>30 μg/ml	Skip next 2 doses and decrease subsequent doses by 50%; recheck serum theophylline level
Too low	7.5–10 μg/ml	Increase dose by about 25%†; recheck serum theophylline concentration after 3 days and then at 6- to 12-month intervals*

Dosage Adjustment After Serum Theophylline Measurement—cont'd

If Serum Level of Theophylline Is	Serum Level	Directions
	5–7.5 μg/ml	Increase dose by about 25% to the nearest dose increment†; recheck serum theophylline level for guidance in further dosage adjustment (another increase will probably be needed, but this provides a safety check)

*Finer adjustments in dosage may be needed for some patients.
†Dividing the daily dose into 3 doses administered at 8-hour intervals may be indicated if symptoms occur repeatedly at the end of a dosing interval.
From Weinberger M, Hendeles L. Practical guide to using theophylline. J Respir Dis 1981;27:12–27.

Dosage in Children <1 Year of Age: Dosage of theophylline in children <1 year of age, particularly in premature and term neonates, has not been well established and must be carefully individualized. Elimination of the drug in children <1 year of age, especially in neonates, generally appears to be reduced. Because of a lack of adequate studies, theophylline is not labeled for use in children <6 months of age. Because of potential toxic effects, use of the drug in children <1 year of age should be carefully considered; if the drug is used, the initial and maintenance dosages (particularly the latter) should be conservative. The recommended oral or IV loading dose of theophylline in these children is 1 mg/kg for each 2 μg/ml increase in serum concentration desired. The recommended initial maintenance dosage in premature neonates up to 40 weeks' postconception age (gestational age at birth plus postnatal age) is 1 mg/kg every 12 hours. The recommended initial maintenance dosage in term neonates (at birth or at 40 weeks' postconception age) is 1–2 mg/kg every 12 hours in those ≤4 weeks' postnatal age, 1–2 mg/kg every 8 hours in those 4–8 weeks' postnatal age, and 1–3 mg/kg every 6 hours in those >8 weeks' postnatal age. Some clinicians suggest that higher initial and maintenance dosages may be necessary in premature neonates. The maintenance dose and dosing interval must be guided by monitoring of serum theophylline concentrations. It is recommended that serum theophylline concentrations be maintained at <10 μg/ml in neonates and at <20 μg/ml in older infants. Maintenance dosage should not be exceeded, and therapy with the drug should not be continued unless the drug is well tolerated and clinically beneficial.

COMMON SIDE EFFECTS: GI irritation, CNS stimulation, nausea, vomiting, epigastric pain, abdominal pain and cramps, anorexia. Adverse effects, which are often more severe in children than in adults, include headache, irritability, restlessness, nervousness, insomnia, dizziness, reflex hyperexcitability, and seizures.

SELECTED DRUG INTERACTIONS: Lithium, oral anticoagulants, cimetidine, high-dose allopurinol (e.g., 600 mg daily), propranolol, ciprofloxacin, erythromycin, troleandomycin, rifampin.

CAUTIONS: Theophylline has a low therapeutic index; therefore cautious dosage determination is essential. Theophylline should be administered with caution to young children, neonates, and infants <1 year of age, patients undergoing influenza immunization, and patients with sustained high fever. Because of marked variation in theophylline metabolism in children <6 months of age, the manufacturers recommend that theophylline not be administered to these children. However, the drug has been used effectively in this age group. Specialized references should be consulted for more information.

Ticarcillin–Clavulanic Acid

SYNONYM: Timentin

CLASS: Penicillin

DOSAGE FORM: Injection: 3.1 g vials

SELECTED DOSAGES: Safety and efficacy in children <12 years of age have not been established. However, children 15 months to 12 years of age have received the 30:1 fixed-ratio combination (3 g ticarcillin; 100 mg clavulanic acid) at a dosage of 207 mg of ticarcillin per kilogram daily in divided doses every 6 hours for the treatment of mild to moderate infections. For the treatment of severe infection, these children have received a dosage of 310 mg of ticarcillin per kilogram daily in divided doses every 4–6 hours. The drug has been used in a limited number of neonates and children <12 years of age without unusual adverse effects. Safety and efficacy of ticarcillin disodium alone and of clavulanate potassium used in combination with amoxicillin have been established in neonates and children.

COMMON SIDE EFFECTS: Rash and urticaria (1.6%), diarrhea, loose stools.

CAUTIONS: The drug shares the toxic potential of the penicillins, including the risk of hypersensitivity reactions. The usual precautions of penicillin therapy should be observed.

Timentin: See ticarcillin–clavulanic acid.

TMP-SMX: See trimethoprim-sulfamethoxazole.

Tobramycin

SYNONYM: Nebcin

CLASS: Aminoglycoside

DOSAGE FORM:
Injection: 10 mg/ml, 40 mg/ml

Powder: 1.2 g

SELECTED DOSAGES: Tobramycin is administered by IM injection or IV infusion. For IV infusion in pediatric patients, the volume of infusion solution depends on the patient's needs but should be sufficient to allow an infusion period of 20–60 minutes. The usual dosage recommended by the manufacturer for children and infants >1 week of age with normal renal function is 3 mg/kg daily, given in equally divided doses at 8-hour intervals. In life-threatening infections, up to 5 mg/kg may be administered daily in 3 or 4 equally divided doses; dosage should be reduced to 3 mg/kg daily as soon as clinically indicated. Dosage in neonates ≤1 week of age should not exceed 4 mg/kg daily, given in equally divided doses at 12-hour intervals. However, some clinicians recommend 5–7.5 mg/kg daily, given in equally divided doses at 12-hour intervals in neonates. Whenever possible, and especially in patients with renal impairment, peak and trough serum concentrations should be determined periodically and dosage should be adjusted to maintain desired serum concentrations. In general, desirable peak serum concentrations are 4–10 μg/ml, and trough concentrations of the drug should not exceed 1–2 μg/ml. An increased risk of toxic effects may be associated with prolonged peak concentrations >10–12 μg/ml and/or troughs >2 μg/ml.

COMMON SIDE EFFECTS: Ototoxic and nephrotoxic effects.

SELECTED DRUG INTERACTIONS: Neurotoxic, ototoxic, or nephrotoxic drugs, general anesthetics and neuromuscular blocking agents, neomycin, nonsteroidal anti-inflammatory agents.

CAUTIONS: Ototoxic and nephrotoxic effects are the most serious adverse effects of therapy. Aminoglycosides should be used with caution and in reduced dosage in preterm and term neonates <6 weeks of age because of the renal immaturity of these patients and the resulting prolongation of serum half-life of the drugs.

Tofranil: See imipramine hydrochloride.

Trandate: See labetalol hydrochloride.

Trimethoprim-sulfamethoxazole

SYNONYM: Bactrim, Co-trimoxazole, Septra, TMP-SMX

CLASS: Sulfonamide

DOSAGE FORM:
Injection: 80 mg trimethoprim + 400 mg sulfamethoxazole per 5 ml

Suspension: oral, 40 mg trimethoprim + 200 mg sulfamethoxazole per 5 ml

Tablets: (scored) 80 mg trimethoprim + 400 mg sulfamethoxazole

Tablets: double-strength, (scored) 160 mg trimethoprim + 800 mg sulfamethoxazole (Bactrim DS; Septra DS)

SELECTED DOSAGES: The drug is available for oral or IV administration. Mix according to the manufacturer's directions. The IV solution should be infused over 60–90 minutes; rapid or direct IV injection must be avoided. Dosage of co-trimoxazole is expressed in terms of the trimethoprim content of the fixed combination containing 5 mg of sulfamethoxazole to 1 mg of trimethoprim.

Otitis Media, Enteritis Caused by *Shigella flexneri* or *Shigella sonnei,* or Chronic or Recurrent Urinary Tract Infections (UTIs): Children ≥2 months of age: usual oral dosage: trimethoprim (as co-trimoxazole), 7.5–8 mg/kg daily, administered in 2 divided doses every 12 hours. The usual duration of co-trimoxazole therapy is 10–14 days for otitis media or chronic or recurrent UTIs or 5 days for enteritis.

Severe UTIs or Enteritis: As above, in children ≥2 months of age: usual IV dosage: trimethoprim (as co-trimoxazole), 8–10 mg/kg daily, administered in 2–4 equally divided doses every 6, 8, or 12 hours for 5 days in the treatment of enteritis or ≤14 days for severe UTIs. The maximum recommended dosage is 960 mg of trimethoprim (as co-trimoxazole) daily.

***Pneumocystis carinii* Pneumonia:** Children >2 months of age: usual oral dosage of trimethoprim (as co-trimoxazole): 20 mg/kg daily, given in 4 divided doses every 6 hours; the usual IV dosage is 15–20 mg/kg daily, given in 3 or 4 equally divided doses every 6 or 8 hours. The usual duration of therapy for *P. carinii* pneumonia is 14 days. For the prophylaxis of *P. carinii* pneumonia, oral trimethoprim (as co-trimoxazole) dosages of 150 mg/m^2 daily in divided doses have been used in adults and children. This use is not in the current labeling.

COMMON SIDE EFFECTS: Nausea, vomiting, anorexia, rash, urticaria.

SELECTED DRUG INTERACTIONS: Warfarin, phenytoin, methotrexate.

CAUTIONS: The manufacturers recommend that the drug not be used in infants <2 months of age. Commercially available preparations contain benzyl alcohol, which has been associated with toxic effects in neonates. Safety and efficacy of repeated courses in children <2 years of age, except those with documented *P. carinii* infections, have not been fully evaluated. The drug should be used with caution in children who have the fragile X chromosome in association with mental retardation, because folate depletion may worsen the psychomotor regression associated with the disorder.

Tylenol: See **acetaminophen.**

Unipen: See nafcillin.

Uniphyl: See theophylline.

Valium: See diazepam.

Valproic Acid

SYNONYM: Depakene

CLASS: Anticonvulsant agent

DOSAGE FORM:
Capsules: 250 mg

Liquid: as the sodium salt, equivalent to 250 mg/5 ml of the acid

SELECTED DOSAGES: A therapeutic range of 50–100 μg/ml has been suggested. The manufacturers state that the usual initial dosage of valproic acid for adults and children is 15 mg/kg daily. Dosage may be increased by 5–10 mg/kg daily at weekly intervals until seizures are controlled or until adverse effects prevent further increases in dosage. The manufacturers state that the maximum recommended dosage is 60 mg/kg daily. To prevent adverse GI effects, the manufacturers state that the drug should be administered in 2 or more divided doses when the dosage exceeds 250 mg daily.

COMMON SIDE EFFECTS: The frequency of adverse effects (particularly hepatic effects) may be dose related. The benefit of improved seizure control, which may accompany higher dosages, should therefore be weighed carefully against the risk of adverse effects. Nausea, vomiting, indigestion, sedation, drowsiness, muscular weakness, enuresis, fatigue.

SELECTED DRUG INTERACTIONS: CNS depressants and anticonvulsants, monoamine oxidase (MAO) inhibitors, aspirin, warfarin.

CAUTIONS: Children <2 years of age, especially those receiving multiple anticonvulsants or those with congenital metabolic disorders, severe seizure disorders accompanied by mental retardation, or organic brain disease, have a considerably increased risk of having a fatal hepatotoxic reaction, in comparison with older patient groups. In children >2 years of age, the frequency

of fatal hepatotoxic reactions decreases considerably in progressively older patient groups.

Vancocin: See vancomycin hydrochloride.

Vancoled: See vancomycin hydrochloride.

Vancomycin Hydrochloride

SYNONYM: Vancocin, Vancoled

CLASS: Antibiotic

DOSAGE FORM:
Capsules: 125 mg, 250 mg

Injection: 500 mg, 1 g vial

Solution: oral, 1 g/bottle

SELECTED DOSAGES: Numerous dosage regimens have been suggested for pediatric patients, particularly neonates and young infants.

Potentially Life-Threatening Infections: For neonates and young infants with normal renal function, the manufacturers recommend an initial IV dose of 15 mg/kg, followed by 10 mg/kg every 12 hours in neonates <8 days of age and 10 mg/kg every 8 hours for infants 8 days to 1 month of age; close monitoring of serum vancomycin concentrations may be warranted in these patients. For older children with normal renal function, the manufacturers recommend an IV dosage of 40 mg/kg daily, given in divided doses. Alternatively, for older children, some clinicians suggest an IV dosage of 1.2 g/m^2 daily, given in divided doses. For specific information on other pediatric dosage regimens, clinicians should consult published protocols and specialized references.

COMMON SIDE EFFECTS: Ototoxic and nephrotoxic effects.

SELECTED DRUG INTERACTIONS: Use of ototoxic and nephrotoxic drugs may result in additive toxic effects (aminoglycosides, amphotericin B, bacitracin, cisplatin, colistin, polymyxin B) should be avoided, if possible.

CAUTIONS: Vancomycin should be used with caution in premature neonates and young infants because of the renal immaturity of these patients and the potential for increased serum concentrations of the drug. Close monitoring of serum vancomycin concentrations may be warranted in neonates and young infants. Concomitant administration of vancomycin and anesthetic agents in children has been associated with erythema and histamine-like flushing. The occurrence of infusion-related adverse effects may be minimized by infusing vancomycin over a period of at least 1 hour before induction of anesthesia.

Vasotec: See **enalapril.**

Ventolin: See **albuterol.**

Verapamil

SYNONYM: Calan, Isoptin

CLASS: Cardiac drug

DOSAGE FORM:
Injection: 5 mg/2 ml

Tablets: (scored) 80 mg, 120 mg (sustained release) 180 mg SR, 240 mg SR

SELECTED DOSAGES:

Supraventricular Tachyarrhythmias: Children <1 year of age: usual initial IV dose of verapamil: 0.75–2 mg (0.1–0.2 mg/kg). In children 1–15 years of age, the usual initial IV dose is 2–5 mg (0.1–0.3 mg/kg), not to exceed 5 mg. The initial pediatric dose may be repeated once after 30 minutes if an adequate response is not achieved. In children 1–15 years of age, the second dose should not exceed 10 mg. Continuous ECG monitoring is especially important during IV administration of the drug in children <1 year of age.

COMMON SIDE EFFECTS: Constipation, nausea, dyspepsia, dizziness, abdominal discomfort, headache, fatigue, bradycardia.

SELECTED DRUG INTERACTIONS: Protein-bound drugs, beta-adrenergic blocking agents, digoxin (may increase serum digoxin concentrations by 50–75% during first week of therapy), hypotensive agents, antiarrhythmic agents, carbamazepine, rifampin, cimetidine, lithium, flecainide, cyclosporine, phenobarbital.

CAUTIONS: Controlled studies with verapamil in children have not been performed to date, but experience in using IV verapamil in more than 250 children (about 50% were <12 months of age and 25% were neonates) indicates that the drug produces effects similar to those in adults. Rarely, severe adverse hemodynamic effects have occurred after IV administration of verapamil in neonates and infants, and the drug should be used with caution in this age group. Safety and efficacy of conventional and extended-release tablets of the drug in children <18 years of age have not been established.

Vibramycin: See **doxycycline.**

Vistaril: See **hydroxyzine.**

Wymox: See **amoxicillin.**

Xylocaine: See **lidocaine.**

Zovirax: See **acyclovir.**

Clinical Tables

1. Allergy, emergency and adjuvant drugs for treatment of physical allergy
2. Allergic rhinitis, environmental considerations
3. Antiarrhythmic drug dosages
4. Anticonvulsants, side effects of commonly used anticonvulsants
5. Antihistamines, classification of commonly used antihistamines
6. Arthritis, drug therapy for chronic childhood arthritis
7. Asthma, dosages for therapy in childhood asthma
8. Asthma, dosages for drug in acute exacerbations of asthma in children
9. Body Surface Area, derivation of body surface area from weight
10. Bone and Joint Infection, commonly used antibiotics for infants and children in bone and joint infections
11. Bronchopulmonary dysplasia, drugs commonly used in the treatment of bronchopulmonary dysplasia
12. Caloric Content of Some Infant Foods
13. Caloric Expenditure and maintenance fluid requirement in children calculated from weight
14. Chlamydia Infection, recommended treatment regimens for incubating and established chlamydial infections
15. Coagulation Deficiencies, products used in coagulation deficiencies
16. Cold Medicines, classification of over the counter cold medicines
17. Diabetic Ketoacidosis, fluid and electrolyte requirements in diabetic ketoacidosis
18. Drug Reactions, Adverse; mechanisms of pharmacologic adverse drug reactions
19. Drug Reactions, Adverse; mechanisms of non-pharmacologic adverse drug reactions
20. Drug Reactions, Adverse; patients at risk for adverse drug reactions
21. Dysmenorrhea; prostaglandin synthetase inhibitors effective in the treatment of primary dysmenorrhea
22. Electrolyte Composition of Commonly Used Oral Solutions
23. Electrolyte Content of Major Body Fluids
24. Empyema, a guide to antimicrobial therapy of bacterial pleurisy and empyema
25. Endocarditis, American Heart Association recommendations for prophylaxis of endocarditis
26. Endocarditis, recommended therapeutic regimens for endocarditis
27. Estrogens, suggested estrogen replacement regimens
28. Factor VIII Concentrates, guidelines for continuous infusion of Factor VIII concentrates

TABLE 1. Emergency and Adjuvant Drugs for Treatment of Physical Allergy

Drug Type	Drug (Trade Name)	Usual Children's Dosage
Sympathomimetics and β-agonists	Epinephrine hydrochloride 1:1000 (Adrenalin)	0.1-0.3 ml/dose SC (0.005-0.01 ml/kg/dose)
	Epinephrine hydrochloride 1:1000 (Adrenalin) in EpiPen and EpiPen Jr. (Center Laboratories)	0.3 and 0.15 ml (EpiPen and EpiPen Jr., respectively) in automatic doser
	Epinephrine 1:200 in thioglycolate (Sus-Phrine)	0.05-0.15 ml/dose SC (0.005 ml/kg/dose)
	Epinephrine hydrochloride 1:1000 (Adrenalin) in Ana-Kit (Hollister-Stier)	0.3 ml/dose; 2 doses possible
	Albuterol (Proventil, Ventolin)	MDI: 1-2 puffs by inhalation 3 × daily or 2-4 mg 3 × daily; syrup: 1 tsp (2 mg) 3-4 × daily in children 6-14 yr; 0.1 mg/kg 3 × daily in children 2-6 yr

	Metaproterenol (Alupent, Metaprel)	MDI: 1-3 puffs by inhalation—not recommended, but used, in children < 12 yr; syrup: 1 tsp (10 mg/5 ml) 3-4 × daily in children 6-9 yr
		Limited published experience in children < 6, but 1.3-2.5 mg/kg/dose 3 × daily well tolerated
	Terbutaline (Bricanyl, Brethine)	2.5-5.0-mg tablet 3 × daily; not recommended for children < 12 yr
Methylxanthine	Theophylline (Slo-bid 50, 100, 200 mg) (Theo-Dur 100, 200, 300 mg)	Therapeutic blood levels; safe therapeutic blood level approx. 10 μg/ml
Anti-inflammatory	Prednisone (Prednisone 5 mg)	As needed
	Cromolyn sodium (Intal)	MDI: 2-3 puffs by inhalation (800 μg per puff) 10-30 minutes before exercise)

Abbreviations: SC, subcutaneous; MDI, metered-dose inhaler.

TABLE 2. Environmental Considerations in Allergic Rhinitis

Examples of Factors Meriting Consideration	Reasons for Consideration
HOME CONSTRUCTION	
Heating system	
Radiator	
Forced air	Possibility for central filtering of forced air systems
Wood	Pollutants from wood stoves
Baseboard	Poor air circulation and mold growth from noncirculating baseboard heat
Humidity	More humid, greater likelihood of dust mite and mold
CLEANING REGIMEN	
Ownership of vacuum cleaner	
Frequency of dusting and vacuuming	May influence dust mite population in the home
Frequency of cleaning drapery and carpet	

HOUSEHOLD CONTENTS	
Age of carpeting and furnishings	The older these items, the more likely they are as sources of dust mites
Quantity of overstuffed articles	
Pets	Source of animal allergies
BEDROOM	
Carpeting, window coverings	Dust mite likely in carpets, overstuffed mattresses, and furniture
Mattress	
Bedding materials	Feathers in bedding attract dust mites and are allergens themselves
Stuffed toys	
AMBIENT AIR QUALITY	
Exposure to tobacco smoke	Pollutants and irritants
Exposure to wood stove	

From Shapiro GG: Allergic rhinitis due to inhalant factors. *In* Rohel RR (ed): Conn's Current Therapy; Philadelphia, WB Saunders Co, p 644, 1988.

TABLE 3. Antiarrhythmic Drug Dosages

Adenosine	50-250 μg/kg rapid IV
Esmolol	500 μg/kg IV over 5 minutes, then 200-500 μg/kg/minute infusion IV
Digoxin (Lanoxin)	Oral digitalization 20-50 μg/kg given ½, ¼, ¼ every 8 hours over first 24 hours
Propranolol	2-8 mg/kg/day p.o. in 4 doses; 1 dose per day of long-acting form
Atenolol	1-2 mg/kg/day p.o. in 1 dose
Phenytoin	3-5 mg/kg/day p.o. in 1 or 2 doses; always use infatabs; maintain serum concentrations >10 <20 μg/ml
Lidocaine	1 mg/kg rapidly IV; maintain 30-50 mg/kg/minute
Procainamide	1 mg/kg IV every 5 minutes × 15 for loading; then maintain 30-50 mg/kg/minute
Flecainide	100-175 mg/M^2/day p.o. divided in 2 doses
Amiodarone	10 mg/kg/day p.o. × 10 days, then 5 mg/kg/day in 1 dose

TABLE 4. Side Effects of Commonly Used Anticonvulsants

Drug	Predictable	Idiosyncratic
Carbamazepine	Diplopia Dizziness Drowsiness Nausea Headache Hyponatremia	Agranulocytosis Lupus-like rash Aplastic anemia Pseudolymphoma Hepatotoxicity Photosensitivity Stevens-Johnson syndrome
Ethosuximide	Anorexia Nausea Vomiting Agitation Drowsiness Lethargy	Rash-erythema multiforme Lupus-like syndrome Stevens-Johnson syndrome Agranulocytosis Aplastic anemia Dystonia
Phenobarbital	Sedation Depression Distractibility Poor memory Hypocalcemia Osteomalacia Irritability	Rash Toxic epidermal necrolysis Hepatic toxicity
Phenytoin	Ataxia Gum hypertrophy Nausea Coarse facies Vomiting Hirsuitism Anorexia Megaloblastic anemia Drowsiness Hypocalcemia Nystagmus Osteomalacia Mental slowing	Blood dyscrasias Lupus-like syndrome Rash Peripheral neuropathy Hepatotoxicity Stevens-Johnson syndrome
Primidone	Nausea Vomiting Weakness Dizziness Diplopia Nystagmus Psychosis Hypocalcemia Osteomalacia Anemia	Rash Agranulocytosis Thrombocytopenia Lupus-like syndrome

Table continued on the following page

TABLE 4. Side Effects of Commonly Used Anticonvulsants *Continued*

Drug	Predictable	Idiosyncratic
Valproate	Anorexia Tremor Sedation Nausea Vomiting Hair loss Drowsiness Weight gain	Acute pancreatitis Hyperammonemia Acute liver toxicity Encephalopathy Rash Thrombocytopenia Neutropenia
Clonazepam	Drowsiness Ataxia Behavior disturbance Increased salivation	Rash Leukopenia Thrombocytopenia

TABLE 5. Classification of Commonly Used Antihistamines

Class	Generic Name	Trade Name	Suggested Dose for Children (mg/kg/24 hr)	Suggested Dose for Adults
Ethanolamine	Diphenhydramine hydrochloride	Benadryl	5.0	25-50 mg q.i.d.
	Carbinoxamine maleate	Clistin	0.8	4-8 mg q.i.d.
Ethylenediamine	Tripelennamine hydrochloride	PBZ	5.0	25-50 mg q.i.d.
Alkylamine	Chlorpheniramine maleate	Chlor-Trimeton Teldrin	0.35	4 mg q.i.d.
	Brompheniramine maleate	Dimetane	0.35	4 mg q.i.d.
	Triprolidine hydrochloride	Actidil	0.18	2.5 q.i.d.
Phenothiazine	Promethazine hydrochloride	Phenergan	0.5	12.5-25 mg q.i.d.
	Methdilazine	Tacaryl	0.3	16-32 mg q.i.d. (as b.i.d. or q.i.d.)
Piperazine	Hydroxyzine hydrochloride	Atarax, Vistaril, Durrax	2.0	10-20 mg q.i.d.
Piperidine	Cyproheptadine hydrochloride	Periactin	0.25	4-20 mg q.i.d.
Miscellaneous	Terfenadine	Seldane	—	60 mg b.i.d.
	Astemizole	Himanal	—	10 mg q.d.

From Shapiro GG: Allergic rhinitis due to inhalant factors. *In* Rohel RR (ed): Conn's Current Therapy; Philadelphia, WB Saunders Co, p 646, 1988.

TABLE 6. Drug Therapy for Chronic Childhood Arthritis

	Size (mg/tab)	Schedule	Dose (mg/kg/day)	Maximum Amount (mg/day)
NONSTEROIDAL ANTI-INFLAMMATORY DRUGS (NSAIDs)				
Salicylate preparations				
Acetylsalicylate (aspirin)	81,325	q.i.d.	60-100 to achieve	
ZORprin	800	b.i.d.	serum level of	
Choline Mg (Trilisate)	500*	t.i.d.	20-25 mg/dl	
Choline Salicylate (Arthropan)	650*	t.i.d.		
Nonsalicylate NSAIDs approved for children				
Tolmetin sodium (Tolectin)	200, 400	t.i.d.	15-30	2000
Naproxen (Naprosyn)	250, 375, 500	b.i.d.	10-20	750
Naproxen liquid	125*	b.i.d. or t.i.d.	10-15	750

NSAIDs not approved for use in children				
Indomethacin (Indocin)	25, 75SR	b.i.d., t.i.d., or q.i.d.	1-3	200
Ibuprofen (Motrin, Advil)	200, 300, 400	q.i.d.	30-70	2400
Fenoprofen Calcium (Nalfon)	200, 300, 600	q.i.d.	40-50	3200
Meclofenamate Sodium (Meclomen)	50, 100	t.i.d.	4-6	300
Sulindac (Clinoril)†	150, 200	b.i.d.	4-6	400
Piroxicam (Feldene)†	10, 20	o.d.	0.5	20
Diclofenac (Voltaren)†	25, 50, 75	b.i.d.	2-3	100-200
SLOW-ACTING ANTIRHEUMATIC DRUGS (SAARDs)				
Gold salts				
Myochrysine, Salgenol	3	Every week (IM)	0.5-1‡	25-50§
Auranofin (Ridaura)		o.d.	0.1	
Hydroxychloroquine (Plaquenil)	200	o.d.	7.0	300
Methotrexate	2.5	Every week (IM or p.o.)	0.1-0.3‡	20-25§

*mg/5 ml.
†Not tested in children.
‡mg/kg/week.
§per week.
Abbreviations: o.d., once a day; b.i.d., twice a day; t.i.d., three times a day; q.i.d., four times a day; IM, intramuscularly; Mg, magnesium.

TABLE 7. Dosages for Therapy in Childhood Asthma

Drug	Mode of Administration	Dosage
B_2-AGONISTS		
Inhaled	Metered-dose inhaler	2 puffs q 4-6 hours
Examples: albuterol, metaproterenol, bitolterol, terbutaline, pirbuteral	Dry powder inhaler	1 capsule q 4-6 hours
	Nebulizer solution*	Albuterol: 5 mg/ml; 0.1-0.15 mg/kg in 2 ml of saline q 4-6 hours, maximum 5.0 mg
		Metaproterenol: 50 mg/ml; 0.25-0.50 mg/kg in 2 ml of saline q 4-6 hours, maximum 15.0 mg
Oral		
Liquids		
Albuterol		0.1-0.15 mg/kg q 4-6 hours
Metaproterenol		0.3-0.5 mg/kg q 4-6 hours
Tablets		
Albuterol		2- or 4-mg tablet q 4-6 hours; 4-mg sustained-release tablet q 12 hours
Metaproterenol		10- or 20-mg tablet q 4-6 hours
Terbutaline		2.5- or 5.0-mg tablet q 4-6 hours
CROMOLYN SODIUM		
Inhaled	Metered-dose inhaler	1 mg/puff; 2 puffs b.i.d.-q.i.d.
	Dry powder inhaler	20 mg/capsule; 1 capsule b.i.d.-q.i.d.
	Nebulizer solution	20 mg/2-ml ampule; 1 ampule b.i.d.-q.i.d.

THEOPHYLLINE	
Liquid	Dosage to achieve serum concentration of 5-15 μg/ml
Tablets, capsules	
Sustained-release tablets, capsules	
CORTICOSTEROIDS	
Inhaled†	
Beclomethasone	42 μg/puff; 2-4 puffs b.i.d.-q.i.d.
Triamcinolone	100 μg/puff; 2-4 puffs b.i.d.-q.i.d.
Flunisolide	250 μg/puff; 2-4 puffs b.i.d.
Oral‡	
Liquids	
Prednisone	5 mg/5 ml
Prednisolone	5 mg/5 ml
	15 mg/5 ml
Tablets	
Prednisone	1, 2.5, 5, 10, 25, 50 mg
Prednisolone	5 mg
Methylprednisolone	2, 4, 8, 16, 24, 32 mg

*Premixed solutions are available. It is suggested that the per-kilogram dosage recommendations be followed.

†Consider use of spacer devices to minimize local adverse effects.

‡For acute exacerbations, doses of 1-2 mg/kg in single or divided doses are used initially and then modified. Reassess in 3 days, as only a short burst may be needed. There is no need to taper a short (3- to 5-day) course of therapy. If therapy extends beyond this period, it may be appropriate to taper the dosage. For chronic dosage, the lowest possible alternate-day morning dosage should be established.

TABLE 8. Dosages for Drugs in Acute Exacerbations of Asthma in Children

Drug	Available Form	Dosage	Comment
INHALED β_2-AGONIST			
Albuterol			
Metered-dose inhaler	90 μg per puff	2 inhalations every 5 minutes for total of 12 puffs, with monitoring of PEFR or FEV_1 to document response	If not improved, switch to nebulizer. If improved, decrease to 4 puffs every hour.
Nebulizer solution	0.5% (5 mg/ml)	0.1-0.15 mg/kg/dose up to 5 mg every 20 minutes for 1-2 hr (minimum dose 1.25 mg/dose) 0.5 mg/kg/hr by continuous nebulization (maximum dose 15 mg/hr)	If improved, decrease to 1-2 hr. If not improved, use by continuous inhalation.
Metaproterenol			
Metered-dose inhaler	650 μg per puff	2 inhalations	Frequent high-dose administration has not been evaluated. Metaproterenol is not interchangeable with β_2-agonists albuterol and terbutaline.
Nebulizer solution	5% (50 mg/ml)	0.1-0.3 cc (5-15 mg). Do not exceed 15 m	
	0.6% unit dose vial of 2.5 ml (15 mg)	As above 5-15 mg. Do not exceed 15 mg	

Terbutaline			
Metered-dose inhaler	200 μg per puff	2 inhalations every 5 minutes for a total of 12 puffs	
Injectable solution used in nebulizer	0.1% (1 mg/1 ml) solution in 0.9% NaCl solution for injection Not FDA-approved for inhalation		Not recommended because not available as nebulizer solution. Offers no advantage over albuterol, which is available as nebulizer solution.
SYSTEMIC β-AGONIST			
Epinephrine Hydrochloride	1:1000 (1 mg/ml)	0.01 mg/kg up to 0.3 mg subcutaneously every 20 minutes for 3 doses	Inhaled β_2-agonist preferred
Terbutaline	(0.1%) 1 mg/ml solution for injection in 0.9% NaCl.	Subcutaneous 0.01 mg/kg up to 0.3 mg every 2-6 hr as needed. Intravenous 10 μg/kg over 10 minutes loading dose. Maintenance: 0.4 μg/kg/minute. Increase as necessary by 0.2 μg/kg/minutes and expect to use 3-6 μg/kg/minute	Inhaled β_2-agonist preferred

Table continued on the following page

TABLE 8. Dosages for Drugs in Acute Exacerbations of Asthma in Children *Continued*

Drug	Available Form	Dosage	Comment
METHYLXANTHINES			
Theophylline	Aminophylline (80% anhydrous theophylline)	Loading dose*: If theophylline concentration known: every 1 mg/kg aminophylline will give 2 μg/ml increase in concentration	
		Loading dose*: If theophylline concentration unknown:	
		—No previous theophylline: 6 mg/kg aminophylline	
		—Previous theophylline: 3 mg/kg aminophylline	
		Constant infusion rates*: Infusion rates to obtain a mean steady-state concentration of 15 μg/ml:	
		Age	
		1-6 months	0.5 mg/kg/hr aminophylline
		6 months-1 year	1.0 mg/kg/hr aminophylline
		1-9 years	1.5 mg/kg/hr aminophylline
		10-16 years	1.2 mg/kg/hr aminophylline

TABLE 9. Estimation of Body Surface Area from Weight

Weight (kg)	Factor × Weight	+ Factor	Example
0-5	0.05	0.05	2 kg, BSA = 0.05 × 2 + 0.05 = 0.15 m^2
5-10	0.04	0.10	9 kg, BSA = 0.04 × 9 + 0.10 = 0.46 m^2
10-20	0.03	0.20	14 kg, BSA = 0.03 × 14 + 0.20 = 0.66 m^2
20-40	0.02	0.40	37 kg, BSA = 0.02 × 37 + 0.40 = 1.14 m^2

Abbreviation: BSA, body surface area.

TABLE 10. Commonly Used Antibiotics for Infants and Children in Bone and Joint Infection

Antibiotic	Intravenous Dosage	Oral Dosage	Maximum
Ampicillin	100-200 mg/kg/24 hr q 6 hr	—	12 g/day
Amoxicillin	—	25-50 mg/kg/24 hr q 8 hr	
Cefazolin	50-100 mg/kg/24 hr q 8 hr	—	6 g/day
Cefotaxime	100-200 mg/kg/24 hr q 6 hr	—	
Cefuroxime	75-150 mg/kg/24 hr q 8 hr	—	6 g/day
Cephalexin	—	100 mg/kg/24 hr q 6 hr	4 g/day
Chloramphenicol	75 mg/kg/24 hr q 6 hr	50-75 mg/kg/24 hr q 6 hr	
Clindamycin	25-40 mg/kg/24 hr q 8 hr	10-30 mg/kg/24 hr q 8 hr	
Dicloxacillin	—	50-75 mg/kg/24 hr q 6 hr	
Gentamicin	6.0-7.5 mg/kg/24 hr q 8 hr	—	
Oxacillin	150-200 mg/kg/24 hr q 6 hr	—	
Vancomycin	40 mg/kg/24 hr q 6 hr	—	

TABLE 11. Drugs Commonly Used in the Treatment of Bronchopulmonary Dysplasia

Drug	Dosage
DIURETICS	
Furosemide	0.5-2.0 mg/kg/dose IV, IM, p.o. q 12 hours (give only once daily in infants <31 weeks' postnatal corrected gestational age because plasma half-life may be up to 24 hours)
Chlorothiazide	5-20 mg/kg per dose p.o. q 12 hours (May give q.o.d. to prevent electrolyte imbalance)
Spironolactone	0.9-1.5 mg/kg per dose p.o. q 12 hours (May give q.o.d. to prevent electrolyte imbalance)
BRONCHODILATORS	
Aminophylline	Loading dose: 5-7 mg/kg per dose IV Maintenance dose: 1.25-2.5 mg/kg per dose IV q 8-12 hours
Metaproterenol	0.3-0.5 mg/kg per dose p.o. q 8 hours
Albuterol	0.02-0.04 ml/kg per dose (aerosol) 0.5% solution (diluted to 1.5-2.0 ml with normal saline solution)
STEROIDS	
Dexamethasone*	0.5 mg/kg/day IV, p.o. divided q 12 hours for 3 days; decrease to 0.3 mg/kg/day for 3 days; decrease by 10% every 3 days; at 0.1 mg/kg per dose, give alternate-day therapy for 1 week, then discontinue

*See Cummings et al. N Engl J Med 320:1505-1510, 1989.

Abbreviations: q, every; q.o.d., every other day; p.o., by mouth.

TABLE 12. Caloric Content of Some Infant Foods

Type	Kilocalories per Serving (~3 Ounces)
Breast milk or formula	60 (20 kcal/ounce)
Infant cereal with formula	110
Infant cereal with water	50
Infant cereal in jars	55-70
Vegetables	25-70
Fruits and juices	40-80
Meats	90-135
Mostly meat dinners	75-105
Whole cow's milk	57 (19 kcal/ounce)
2% cow's milk	45 (15 kcal/ounce)
Skim cow's milk	30 (10 kcal/ounce)

TABLE 13. Calculation of Caloric Expenditure and Maintenance Fluid Requirement Based on Body Weight

Body Weight (kg)	Caloric Expenditure (kcal) and Fluid Requirement (ml)
Up to 10	100 × weight
10-20	1000 + 50 × (weight − 10)
Over 20	1500 + 20 × (weight − 20)

TABLE 14. Recommended Treatment Regimens for Incubating and Established Chlamydial Infection*

Antibiotic	Regimen by Patient's Weight ≥45 kg	<45 kg	Comments
Doxycycline or	100 mg p.o. b.i.d. for 7 days		Tetracyclines are not indicated during pregnancy and for children younger than 8 years of age
Tetracycline	500 mg p.o. q.i.d. for 7 days	40 mg/kg/day in 4 doses for 7 days	
Erythromycin base or	500 mg p.o. q.i.d. for 7 days	40 mg/kg/day in 4 doses for 7 days	Use for pregnant patients and children under 8 years of age
Erythromycin ethylsuccinate	800 mg p.o. q.i.d. for 7 days	40 mg/kg/day in 4 doses for 7 days	

☐ Adapted from the Centers for Disease Control: 1989 Sexually Transmitted Diseases Treatment Guidelines. MMWR 38(suppl 8), 1989; and the American Academy of Pediatrics: 1988 Report of the Committee on Infectious Diseases. Reprinted from Paradise JE: The medical evaluation of the sexually abused child. Pediatr Clin North Am 37(4):839-862, 1990.

**Warning:* These recommendations are not for patients with suspected or definite pelvic inflammatory diseases.

Abbreviations: p.o., orally; b.i.d., twice a day; q.i.d., four times a day.

TABLE 15. Products Used in Coagulation Deficiencies

Product Name	Manufacturer	Method of Viral Depletion/Inactivation	Specific Activity*: Final	Specific Activity*: Discounting Albumin	Hepatitis Safety Studies in Humans: With this Product	Hepatitis Safety Studies in Humans: With Similar Product
RECOMBINANT (R) VIII PRODUCTS						
Recombinate	Baxter	See footnote†	1.65–19	3000+‡	Yes	—
Kogenate	Miles	See footnote§	8–30	3000+‡	Yes	—
IMMUNOAFFINITY PURIFIED FVIII PRODUCTS DERIVED FROM HUMAN PLASMA						
Monoclate P	Armour	Pasteurized, 60°C, 10h	@5–10	3000+	Yes (ongoing)	Yes
Hemofil M	Baxter-Hyland	Solvent-detergent (TNBP + Triton X-100, 25°C, ≥10h	@2–11	3000+	Yes(1)	—
Coagulation FVIII, Method M	(Manufactured by Baxter-Hyland for Red Cross)	Solvent-detergent (TNBP + Triton X-100), 25°C, ≥10h	@2–11	3000+	No	Yes(1)
Profilate OSD	Alpha	Solvent-detergent (TNBP + polysorbate 80), 27°C, 6h	@6–10		No	Yes
Koate-HP	Cutter	Solvent-detergent (TNBP + polysorbate 80), ≥24°C, 6h	@9–22	50	No	Yes
NY Blood Center FVIII-SD	NYBC, Melville Biologics	Solvent-detergent (TNBP + cholate), ≥24°C, 6h	@1		Yes(2)	
Humate P	Behringwerke (distrib: Armour)	Heated in solution (pasteurized), 60°C, 10 h	@1–2		Yes(3)	—
Melate SD	NYBC, Melville Biologics	Solvent-detergent (TNBP + polysorbate 80), ≥24°C, 6h	@50–150		No	Yes
COAGULATION FIX PRODUCTS						
AlphaNine	Alpha	Heated in *n*-heptane solution, 60°C, 20h, and affinity chromatography	@84		No	Yes (with HCV transmission in 1980s)
AlphaNine SD	Alpha	TNBP + polysorbate 80, 24°–30°C, >24h, and affinity chromatography	@190		No	Yes

Mononine	Armour	Monoclonal antibody column, sodium thiocyanate, ultra-filtration	160 +	Yes[4]	
FIX COMPLEX CONCENTRATES					
Konyne 80	Cutter	Dry heat, 80°C, 80°C, 72h	Not available	No	Yes[5]
Proplex T	Baxter-Hyland	Dry heat, 68°C, 144h	@47	No	No
Profilnine HT (wet method)	Alpha	Heated in *n*-heptane solution, 60°C, 20h	@4.5	No	Yes[6] (with HCV transmission in 1980s)
Bebulin	Immuno	Vapor heated (10h, 60°C, 1190 mbar pressure plus 1h, 80°C, 1375 mbar	@2	Yes[7]	
ACTIVATED FIX COMPLEX CONCENTRATES					
Autoplex T	Baxter-Hyland	Dry heat, 68°C, 144h	@5	No	No
FEIBA VH	Immuno	Vapor heated (10h, 60°C, 1190 mbar plus 1h, 80°C, 1375 mbar)	@0.8	No	Yes[8]
PORCINE FVIII					
Hyate C	Porton/Speywood	None	>50	No (but no report of transmission of human viruses)	No

*NOTE: The degree of product purity is reflected by the specific activity of FVIII (units/mg protein). Since most FVIII concentrates (including recombinant FVIII) have human serum albumin added as a stabilizer, most persons look at the specific activity discounting albumin. The immunoaffinity purified FVIII preparations are thus often referred to as "ultrapure," or very high purity FVIII.

†The production process for Recombinate contains a number of steps (immunoaffinity chromatography, exposure to virucidal solutions, pasteurization, etc.) that are capable of inactivating or removing viruses. The process has been validated to inactivate or exclude $>1 \times 10^7$ log of model enveloped and nonenveloped viruses.

‡Representative sample from in-process materials prior to addition of albumin.

§The production process for Kogenate combines anion and immunoaffinity chromatography with heat treatment step. This process has been validated for a 12 log reduction of relevant model viruses.

NOTE: References for this table are on page 210.

TABLE 16. Classification of Over-the-Counter Cold Medicines

Class	Examples	Side Effects
Sympathomimetics	Phenylpropanolamine Pseudoephedrine Phenylephrine	Excess stimulation; irritability; hypertension; insomnia
Antihistamines	Ethanolamines (diphenhydramine) Alkylamines (chlorpheniramine, brompheniramine)	Sedation; paradoxical central nervous system stimulation
Expectorants	Guaifenesin	Gastric upset
Cough suppressants	Codeine	Drowsiness; respiratory depression
	Dextromethorphan	Sedation; gastrointestinal upset

TABLE 17. Fluid and Electrolyte Requirements in Diabetic Ketoacidosis

	Maintenance/m²	Deficit Repair/kg
Water	1500 ml	100 ml
Sodium	60 mEq	7-10 mEq
Potassium	50 mEq	5-10 mEq
Chloride	40 mEq	5 mEq
Phosphate	10 mEq	3 mEq

TABLE 18. Mechanisms of Pharmacologic Adverse Drug Reactions

Mechanism	Example
Accentuated dose-related pharmacologic effect	Hypotension during antihypertensive therapy
Dose-related toxic effect	Central nervous system irritability during theophylline therapy
Drug interaction—pharmacokinetic	Reduction of theophylline clearance by erythromycin
Drug interaction—pharmacodynamic	Apnea with combined administration of morphine and diazepam
Toxicity due to altered disposition or elimination due to altered renal or liver function	Digoxin accumulation in renal failure Increased unbound phenytoin during renal failure

TABLE 19. Mechanisms of Non-pharmacologic Adverse Drug Reactions

Mechanism	Example
Idiosyncratic—inapparent feature of patient leading to adverse drug reaction	Hemolysis after exposure to antimalarial drugs in patients with glucose-6-phosphate dehydrogenase deficiency Aspirin-induced bronchospasm Prolonged effect of succinylcholine due to low serum esterase activity Phenytoin hypersensitivity due to probable generation of reactive metabolite that may become a hapten
Allergic/immune-mediated	Penicillin anaphylaxis Serum sickness with sulfonamides Stevens-Johnson syndrome with phenobarbital therapy
Anaphylactoid reactions—release of mediators of anaphylaxis without involvement of IgE	Vancomycin-induced cutaneous flushing Radiologic contrast media reactions

TABLE 20. Patients at Risk for Adverse Drug Reactions

- Patient taking multiple drugs
- Critically ill patients
- Patients with altered renal or liver function
- Patients taking drugs that alter disposition or metabolism of other drugs
- Oncology patients

TABLE 21. Prostaglandin Synthetase Inhibitors Effective in the Treatment of Primary Dysmenorrhea

Drug	Dose
FENAMATES	
Meclofenamate sodium (Meclomen)	100 mg t.i.d.
Mefanamic acid (Ponstel)	500 mg initially, then 250 mg t.i.d.
PROPIONIC ACID DERIVATIVES	
Ibuprofen (Advil, Motrin)	400 mg q.i.d.
Naproxyn sodium (Anaprox DS)	550 mg t.i.d.
Naproxyn (Naprosyn)	500 mg initially, then 250 mg q.i.d.
Ketoprofen (Orudis)	25-50 mg q.i.d.

Abbreviations: t.i.d., three times a day; q.i.d., four times a day.

TABLE 22. Electrolyte Composition of Some Commonly Used Oral Solutions

	Na	K	Cl	Base (mEq/L)
Water	0	0	0	0
Cow's milk	25	35	30	
Breast milk/formula	7	15-20	12	
Carbonated soft drinks	0-10	0-15	0-15	0-15
Kool-Aid	0	0	0	
Apple juice	2	25	0	
Orange juice	0	50	0	50
Pedialyte	45	20	35	
Ricelyte	50	25	45	
Rehydrate	75	20	65	
Gatorade	21	2.5	17	
WHO solution	90	20	80	30

Abbreviations: WHO, World Health Organization.

TABLE 23. Electrolyte Content of Major Body Fluids

Fluid	Na (mEq/L)	K (mEq/L)	Cl (mEq/L)
Gastric	20-80	5-20	100-150
Pancreas, small intestine, bile	120-140	5-15	80-130
Ileum	45-135	3-15	20-115
Diarrhea	10-90	10-80	10-110
Sweat, normal	10-30	3-10	10-35
Sweat, cystic	50-130	5-25	50-110

Abbreviations: Na, sodium; K, potassium; Cl, chloride.

TABLE 24. A Guide to Antimicrobial Therapy of Bacterial Pleurisy and Empyema

Infecting Agent	Drug and Dosage (per kg per day) Route and Duration*
A. Aerobic bacteria	
1. Staphylococci	1. a. Methicillin, 200-400 mg divided in 3-4 doses IV initially; for 3-4 weeks b. Cloxacillin, 100-200 mg divided in 3-6 doses IV initially; for 3-4 weeks
2. *Haemophilus influenzae*	2. a. Ampicillin, 100-200 mg divided in 2-4 doses IV initially; for 1-2 weeks or b. Chloramphenicol, 50-100 mg divided in 4 doses IV initially; for 1-2 weeks or c. Cefuroxime, 75-225 mg divided in 3 doses IV initially; for 1-2 weeks
3. Pneumococcus and streptococci	3. Penicillin G, 50,000-300,000 units divided in 3-4 doses IV or IM; for 7-10 days
4. *Escherichia coli* and *Klebsiella*	4. Gentamicin, 5-7 mg divided in 2-3 doses IV; for 14 days or longer
5. *Pseudomonas*	5. a. Carbenicillin, 100-600 mg divided in 4 doses IV; for 10 days or longer or b. Ticarcillin, 400 mg, divided in 4 doses IV; for 10 days or longer c. Tobramycin, 5-7 mg divided in 2 doses
B. Anaerobic bacteria	
1. *Bacteroides fragilis*	1. Chloramphenicol, same as A.2.b
2. All except *B. fragilis*	2. a. Penicillin G, same as A.3 b. Ampicillin, same as A.2.a

TABLE 25. American Heart Association Recommendations for Prophylaxis of Endocarditis*

Procedure	Antibiotic	Dosage
Dental, oral, upper respiratory tract	Amoxicillin p.o.	50 mg/kg 1 hr before procedure (max 3.0 g) 25 mg/kg 6 hr after procedure (max 1.5 g)
In penicillin-allergic patient	Erythromycin p.o.	20 mg/kg 1 hour before procedure; 10 mg/kg 6 hr after procedure
	or	
	Clindamycin p.o.	10 mg/kg 1 hour before procedure 5 mg/kg 6 hr after procedure
Genitourinary/gastrointestinal	Ampicillin IV	50 mg/kg 30 minutes before procedure (max 2.0 g)
	+	
	Gentamicin IV	2.0 mg/kg 30 minutes before procedure (max 80 mg) Repeat this regimen 8 hr after procedure
In penicillin-allergic patient	Vancomycin IV	20 mg/kg 1 hr before procedure (max 500 mg)
	+	
	Gentamicin IV	2.0 mg/kg 1 hr before (max 80 mg) Repeat this regimen 8 hr after procedure
If low risk†	Amoxicillin p.o.	50 mg/kg 1 hr before procedure (max 3.0 g) 25 mg/kg 6 hr after procedure (max 1.5 g)

*These are the 1990 recommendations, and revisions are made frequently.
†Procedures and lesions are described in American Heart Association recommendations adapted from JAMA 264:2919-2922, 1990. Copyright 1990, American Medical Association.

TABLE 26. Recommended Therapeutic Regimens for Endocarditis

Organism	Sensitivity	Antibiotic (Dosage)	Duration
Streptococci			
On native valve	MIC $<$ 0.1 μg/ml*	Penicillin G (200,000-250,000 units/kg/day IV div q 4 hr) *or*	4 weeks
		Penicillin G (200,000-250,000 units/kg/day IV div q 4 hr) + Gentamicin (1 mg/kg/dose IV q 8 hr)	2 weeks†
	MIC $>$ 0.1 μg/ml	Penicillin G (200,000-250,000 units/kg/day IV) + Gentamicin (1 mg/kg/dose IV q 8 hr)	4 weeks
In penicillin-allergic patient		Vancomycin (40-60 mg/kg/day IV div q 6 hr) + Gentamicin (1 mg/kg/dose IV q 8 hr)	4 weeks
On prosthetic valve		Vancomycin and gentamicin (as in penicillin-allergic patient)	6 weeks
Enterococci		Penicillin G (200,000-250,000 units/kg/day IV div q 4 hr) + Gentamicin (1 mg/kg/dose IV q 8 hr)	6 weeks

Staphylococci	Oxacillin-sensitive	Oxacillin or nafcillin (150-200 mg/kg/day IV div q 6 hr) +	4-6 weeks
		Gentamicin (1 mg/kg/dose IV q 8 hr)	1-2 weeks
		Consider rifampin (20 mg/kg/day p.o. div q 12 hr)‡	2-4 weeks
	Oxacillin-resistant *or* In penicillin-allergic patient	Vancomycin (40-60 mg/kg/day IV div q 6 hr) +	4-6 weeks
		Gentamicin (1 mg/kg/dose IV q 8 hr)	1-2 weeks
		Consider rifampin (20 mg/kg/day p.o. div q 12 hr)	2-4 weeks
Gram-negative organisms		Consult microbiology laboratory sensitivities	6 weeks
Fungi		Amphotericin B 1 mg/kg/dose/day IV + flucytosine 50 mg/kg/day p.o. div q 6 hr	6 weeks minimum
		Surgery	

*Minimum inhibitory concentration to penicillin.

†Consider two additional weeks of treatment with amoxicillin.

‡If slow clinical response or abscess suspected or if coagulase-negative *Staphylococcus* infection of prosthetic valve.

Abbreviations: MIC, minimum inhibitory concentration; IV, intravenous; p.o., by mouth; q, every; hr, hour; div, divided.

TABLE 27. Suggested Estrogen Replacement Regimens

- Conjugated estrogens (Premarin) 0.625-1.25 mg on days 1-25

  plus

  Medroxyprogesterone acetate (Provera) 5-10 mg on days 14-25

  or

- 17β-estradiol (Estrace) 1-2 mg on days 1-25

  plus

  Medroxyprogesterone acetate (Provera) 5-10 mg on days 14-25

  or

- Oral contraceptive (30-35 μg estrogen with nonandrogenic progestin)

TABLE 28. Guidelines for Continuous Infusion of Factor VIII Concentrates

Infuse bolus to increase to desired level (1 unit/kg elevates level by 2%).

Maintain 25%: 1 units/kg/hr.
50%: 2 units/kg/hr.
75%: 3 units/kg/hr.

Dispense factor VIII in batches for 12-hour infusions mixed in 500 or 1000 ml of normal saline.

Assay factor VIII levels once daily to ensure that appropriate level is maintained.

TABLE 29. Factors That May Require Adjustment in Fluid Intake

INCREASED REQUIREMENT
Fever, increase in environmental temperature, radiant heat losses
Open abdominal defect (e.g., omphalocele, gastroschisis)
Phototherapy
Physical activity (e.g., tachypnea, hyperthyroidism)
Prematurity
Third-space losses, including postoperative patients
DECREASED REQUIREMENT
Congestive heart failure
Humidified isolette
Immobilization (e.g., congenital neuromuscular disease, cast placement)
Mechanical ventilation
Pharmacologic neuromuscular blockade
Symptomatic patent ductus arteriosus

TABLE 30. Recommended Baseline Fluid Requirements for Infants (ml/kg/day)

Age	Days 1-2	Days 3-5	Days 10-42	Comments
PRETERM				
<1000 g	90-100	110-≥180	130-160	May lose 7-10% body weight in first week of life; avoid fluid overload contributing to symptoms of patent ductus arteriosus, bronchopulmonary dysplasia, and hyponatremia
>1000 g	80-100	100-140	120-150	
TERM	60-80	80-120	100-150	Baseline insensible losses 20 ml/kg; less transepidermal loss than in premature
SMALL-FOR-GESTATIONAL-AGE	70-90	100-140	120-160	In general, should not lose weight after birth; avoid dehydration, which could worsen the frequently associated polycythemia

TABLE 31. Recommended Treatment Regimens for Incubating and Established Gonococcal Infections*

	Regimen by Patient's Weight		
Antibiotic	**≥45 kg**	**<45 kg**	**Comments**
Amoxicillin† with probenecid	3.0 g p.o. 1.0 g p.o.	50 mg/kg p.o. 25 mg/kg p.o.	Use only when gonococci are known to be penicillin-sensitive; amoxicillin may not treat pharyngeal infection
Ceftriaxone	250 mg IM	125 mg IM	Use when antibiotic sensitivity of organism is unknown
Spectinomycin	2.0 g IM	40 mg/kg IM	Use for patients with penicillin allergy; may not treat incubating syphilis and pharyngeal gonorrhea

**Warning:* Concurrent presumptive treatment for chlamydial infection is recommended. These recommendations are not for patients with suspected or definite pelvic inflammatory disease.

†Other penicillin regimens including benzathine penicillin and penicillin V are not recommended.

Abbreviations: p.o., orally; IM, intramuscularly.

☐ Adapted from the Centers for Disease Control: 1989 Sexually Transmitted Diseases Treatment Guidelines. MMWR 38(suppl 8), 1989; and the American Academy of Pediatrics: 1988 Report of the Committee on Infectious Diseases. Reprinted in Paradise JE: The medical evaluation of the sexually abused child. Pediatr Clin North Am 37(4) 839-862, 1990.

TABLE 32. Griseofulvin Dosage and Therapy

Dosage (7.3 mg/kg/24 hr)		Therapy	
Weight (lb)	**Daily Dosage Range (mg)**	**Site**	**Duration of Therapy**
35-60*	125-187.5	Scalp	4-8 wk
60-100	187-375	Skin	3-4 wk
100-125	317-453	Palms and soles	8-12 wk
		Fingernails	4-9 mo
		Toenails†	6-18 mo

*Dosage has not been established for children 2 years of age or younger.
†Requires an increase in dosage by a factor of 50 to 100 per cent.

TABLE 33. Drugs Used in Head Injury

Name	Dose	Route	Use	Comments
Oxygen	100%	Mask, ET, cannula	Ensure oxygenation	Pulse oximetry helpful
Atropine	0.02 mg/kg	IV, IM, ET, SC	Dry secretions, prevent bradycardia	Minimum dose 0.1 mg
Thiopental	2 mg/kg	IV	Sedation	May depress circulation
Succinylcholine	2 mg/kg (<1 year) 1 mg/kg (>1 year)	IV, IM	Depolarizing paralyzer	Contraindicated in crush injury, burn, hyperkalemia
Vecuronium	0.1 mg/kg	IV	Nondepolarizing paralyzer	May increase intracranial pressure
Pancuronium	0.1 mg/kg	IV	Nondepolarizing paralyzer	Tachycardia
Midazolam	0.2 mg/kg 0.4-6 μ/kg/minute	IV IV infusion	Sedation	
Diazepam	0.2 mg/kg	IV	Sedation anticonvulsant	Respiratory depression
Mannitol (20%)	0.25-2 g/kg	IV	Decrease ICP	Hyperosmolar state
Furosemide	1 mg/kg	IV		
Ethacrynic acid	1 mg/kg	IV		
Pentobarbital	3-5 mg/kg 1-3 mg/kg/hr	IV IV infusion	Decrease ICP	30-40 μg/ml blood level; CNS and circulatory effects
Phenytoin	15-20 mg/kg	IV	Anticonvulsant	Bradycardia

Abbreviations: IV, intravenous (intraosseous); IM, intramuscular; ET, endotracheal; SC, subcutaneous; ICP, intracranial pressure; CNS, central nervous system.

TABLE 34. Diagnosis and Therapy in Chronic Active Hepatitis

Diagnosis	Laboratory Indicator	Therapy
Wilson's disease	Elevated urine copper; low ceruloplasmin	Penicillamine (10-20 mg/kg)
$Alpha_1$-antitrypsin deficiency	ZZ phenotype	Symptomatic Transplantation
Hepatitis B	sAg, cAb, eAg, eAb	Alpha interferon?
Hepatitis C	Hepatitis C Ab	Alpha interferon?
Autoimmune hepatitis	ANA, antiLKM, anti-smooth muscle, IgG	Prednisone (2 mg/kg) ± azathioprine

TABLE 35. Treatment of Hyperkalemia

Agent	Action	Dose
Calcium gluconate (10%)	Counteracts the cardiac effects of potassium	100-200 mg/kg per dose over 30-60 minute
Sodium bicarbonate	Shifts potassium intracellularly	1 mEq/kg per dose over 30-60 minute
Glucose and insulin	Shifts potassium intracellularly	0.5 g/kg of glucose with 0.3 U regular insulin per gram of glucose over 2 hr
Kayexalate	Exchanges potassium for sodium in the gut	1-2 g/kg/day, divided q 6 hr in 70% sorbitol solution (3 ml/g resin) p.o. or nasogastric tube; or as a retention enema in 20% sorbitol solution (5 ml/g resin)

TABLE 36. Therapy of Hyperlipidemia

	Mechanism	% Reduction in Cholesterol	Effect of VLDL	Effect on HDL	Side Effects	Dose
NONPHARMACOLOGIC THERAPY						
AHA Prudent Diet	Limits exogenous cholesterol	10-15%	Decrease	Decrease	—	
Exercise	Improves insulin resistance	Some decrease	Decrease	Increase	—	
Weight loss	Improves insulin resistance	Some decrease	Decrease	Mild increase	—	
PHARMACOLOGIC THERAPY						
Bile acid resins	Accelerates LDL disposal	20-30%	Mild decrease	Mild increase	Epigastric distress, constipation, bloating, interferes with some drug absorption	Up to 24 g/day of cholestyramine in divided doses
Nicotinic acid or niacin	Reduces VLDL and LDL synthesis; increases HDL	25%	50% decrease	30-40% increase	Flushing, headache, tachycardia, GI distress, activation of	Titrate up to 1 g 3 times a day

					peptic ulcer disease and inflammatory bowel disease, hepatic dysfunction	
Probucol	Increases LDL disposal; reduces HDL/LDL ratio	5-15%	—	Decrease	Nausea, diarrhea, flatulence, eosinophilia, hepatic dysfunction, prolong Q-T interval	0.5 g twice a day
Gemfibrozol (Lopid)	Enhances VLDL breakdown and decreased VLDL production	Decrease	40-50% decrease	20-30% increase	Rarely myositis, should not be used in patients with renal disease, cholelithiasis, or liver dysfunction	600 mg twice a day
HMG-CoA reductase inhibitor (Lovastatin)	Inhibits cholesterol synthesis and increases LDL disposal	30-40%	—	—	Elevated liver enzymes, myositis, cataracts in animals	20-40 mg twice a day

Abbreviations: AHA, American Heart Association; HMG-CoA, 3-hydroxy-3-methylglutaryl coenzyme A; LDL, low-density lipoprotein; HDL, high-density lipoprotein; VLDL, very-low-density lipoprotein; GI, gastrointestinal.

TABLE 37. Medications for Treatment of Chronic Hypertension*

Drug	Initial Daily Dose	Maximum Daily Dose	Frequency	Available Formulations
DIURETICS				
Hydrochlorothiazide	1.0 mg/kg (60 mg/m^2)	100 mg	b.i.d.	50 mg/5 ml solution; 25, 50, 100 mg tablets
	3.0 mg/kg (<6 months of age)	37.5 mg	b.i.d.	
Chlorothiazide	20 mg/kg (600 mg/m^2)	1000 mg	b.i.d.	250 mg/5 ml solution; 250, 500 mg tablets
	30 mg/kg (<6 months of age)	375 mg (up to 2 yrs)	b.i.d.	
Furosemide	1-2 mg/kg	320 mg or 4 mg/kg	b.i.d., q.d.	40 mg/5 ml, 10 mg/ml solution; 20, 40, 80 mg tablets
Potassium Sparing				
Spironolactone	1-3 mg/kg	6 mg/kg/24 hr	12-24 hr	25 mg
Triamterene	2-4 mg/kg	4 mg/kg/24 hr	12 hr	50, 100 mg
Metolazone	0.07-0.14 mg/kg	0.3 mg/kg/24 hr	24 hr	2.5, 5, 10 mg
β-ADRENERGIC ANTAGONISTS				
Nonselective				
Propranolol	1-2 mg/kg	8 mg/kg	b.i.d.	20 mg/5 ml solution; 10, 20, 40, 60, 80 mg tablets

Nadolol	40 mg†	640 mg	q.d.	20, 40, 80, 120 mg tablets
Selective				
Atenolol	50 mg†	100 mg	q.d.	25, 50, 100 mg tablets
Metoprolol	100-200 mg†	450 mg	q.d., b.i.d.	50, 100 mg tablets
Acebutolol	200-400 mg†	1200 mg	q.d.	200, 400 mg tablets
α-ADRENERGIC ANTAGONISTS				
Prazosin	1-2 mg	20 mg	b.i.d., t.i.d.	1, 2, 5 mg tablets
COMPLEX ADRENERGIC ANTAGONISTS				
Labetalol	50-100 mg†	1200-2400 mg	b.i.d.	100, 200, 300 mg tablets
CENTRAL SYMPATHOLYTICS				
α-Methyldopa	10 mg/kg (300 mg/m^2)	65 mg/kg (2 g/m^2)	b.i.d., t.i.d., q.i.d.	250 mg/5 ml solution; 125, 250, 500 mg tablets
Clonidine	0.05-0.1 mg tablet	2.4 mg by mouth	b.i.d., t.i.d.	0.1, 0.2, 0.3 mg tablets
	0.1 mg/day patch	0.6 mg by patch	q week	0.1, 0.2, 0.3 mg patches
Guanabenz	0.08-0.2 mg/kg (>12 yr)	64 mg	b.i.d.	4, 8 mg tablets
DIRECT VASODILATORS				
Hydralazine	0.5-1.0 mg/kg (25 mg/m^2)	4-8 mg/kg (200 mg)	t.i.d., q.i.d.	10, 25, 50 mg tablets
Minoxidil	0.1 mg/kg	1 mg/kg (50 mg)	b.i.d., q.d.	2.5, 10 mg tablets

Table continued on following page

TABLE 37. Medications for Treatment of Chronic Hypertension* *Continued*

Drug	Initial Daily Dose	Maximum Daily Dose	Frequency	Available Formulations
CALCIUM CHANNEL BLOCKERS				
Nifedipine	0.25 mg/kg	1-2 mg/kg (180 mg)	t.i.d., q.i.d.	10, 20 mg capsules;
Extended Release		1-2 mg/kg (90 mg)	q.d.	30, 60, 90 mg tablets
Diltiazem	60-120 mg†	360 mg	b.i.d., q.d.	60, 90, 120 mg tablets
Verapamil	120-240 mg†	480 mg	b.i.d., q.d.	120, 240 mg tablets
ANGIOTENSIN-CONVERTING ENZYME INHIBITORS				
Captopril	0.05-0.1 mg/kg	4 mg/kg (200 mg)	b.i.d., t.i.d.	12.5, 25, 50, 100 mg tablets
Enalapril	1.25-2.5 mg†	40 mg	b.i.d., q.d.	2.5, 5, 10, 20 mg tablets
Lisinopril	2.5 mg†	20 mg	b.i.d., q.d.	5, 10, 20, 40 mg tablets

*Additional agents are available; however, not all are listed. The experience with the many new beta-blockers and converting enzyme inhibitors is limited in children.

†Pediatric dose is not established.

TABLE 38. Treatment of Hypertension

Drug	Dose-Route	Comments
Hydralazine	0.1-0.4 mg/kg IV or IM	Dose may be increased and repeated in 10-15 minutes, minimal acute toxicity, less effective as a chronic medication.
Nifedipine	0.25-0.5 mg/kg p.o. or sublingually	Effective orally, but awkward to use because the smallest dosage size is a 10-mg capsule.
Diazoxide	3-5 mg/kg IV	May be given as a bolus (smaller doses) or slow infusion (over 15-20 minutes) to “titrate” blood pressure reduction. Cannot be given as a bolus through a central catheter (arrhythmia risk). Repeated dosing may lead to hyperglycemia.
Labetalol	0.5-3 mg/kg IV	After an initial dose, the blood pressure may be adjusted by a slower continuous infusion.
Sodium nitroprusside	Continuous IV infusion at 0.5-8.0 μg/kg/hr (50 mg in 1000 ml of D_5W = 50 μg/ml	May cause profound, abrupt hypotension; requires continuous careful monitoring. Thiocyanate accumulation may occur and produce toxicity.

TABLE 39. Hypertensive Crises: Blood Pressure Values by Age

Age (Years)	Hypertensive Crises (mm Hg)
<2	145/95
3-5	150/95
6-9	160/100
10-12	165/105
13-15	175/110
16-18	185/120

TABLE 40. Medications for Treatment of Hypertensive Crisis

Drug	Route	Dose	Maximum	Frequency
Sodium nitroprusside	IV	0.5 μg/kg/minute; *Neonate:* 0.3 μg/kg/minute	8.0 μg/kg/minute 6.0 μg/kg/minute	Continuous
Diazoxide	IV	1-3 mg/kg	10 mg/kg/day (600 mg/day)	Rapid push over 1-2 minutes
Labetalol	IV	0.2-0.4 mg/kg (1-3 mg/kg/hr)	3-4 mg/kg/day (300 mg/day)	Bolus (continuous)
Nifedipine	p.o./SL	0.25-0.50 mg/kg; <10 yr, 2.5 mg 11-20 yr, 5 mg; >20 yr, 10 mg	20 mg/dose	30-60 minutes
Minoxidil	p.o.	0.1-0.2 mg/kg	0.5 mg/kg/day (40 mg/day)	2-6 hr
Clonidine	p.o.	0.05-0.10 mg	2.4 mg/day	1-2 hr
Hydralazine	IV/IM	0.2 mg/kg	0.6 mg/kg/dose (20 mg/dose)	2-6 hr
Phentolamine	IV	0.1-0.2 mg/kg (2-10 mg)	10 mg/dose	5-15 minutes
Adjunct drugs for hypertensive crisis (Diuretics)				
Furosemide	IV	1-6 mg/kg		If no response, repeat in 1 hr at higher dose
Ethacrynic acid	IV	0.5-1.5 mg/kg		If no response, repeat in 1 hr at higher dose

Abbreviations: IV, intravenous; IM, intramuscular; p.o., oral; SL, sublingual.

TABLE 41. Calcium and Magnesium Supplementation in Hypocalcemia and Tetany

Supplement	Dosage
Calcium carbonate (40% elemental calcium)	500 mg tab = 200 mg calcium
Calcium chloride 10%	IV 100 mg/kg per dose, 200-500 mg/kg/day IV
	p.o. Infant: 400-800 mg/kg/day q 6 hr
	Child: 200-500 mg/kg/day q 6 hr
	1.36 mEq elemental Ca/ml
	IV 20 mg/kg per dose
Calcium gluconate 10%	0.45 mEq elemental calcium/ml
Dihydrotachysterol	0.025-0.05 mg/kg/day
25-Hydroxyvitamin D_3	0.7-2.8 mg/kg/day
1,25-Dihydroxyvitamin D_3	20-50 mg/kg/day
Calcium-enriched milk	Add 400-800 mg elemental calcium to 1 L breast milk or Similac PM 60/40
Magnesium sulfate 10%	100 mg/ml = 0.8 mEq/ml
Magnesium sulfate 50%	500 mg/ml = 4.0 mEq/ml
Magnesium gluconate tablets	500 mg = 4 mEq
Magnesium gluconate syrup	54 mg/5 ml

TABLE 42. Laboratory Data and Treatment of the Four Types of Hyponatremia

	Laboratory Data	Treatment
Water intoxication	Low sp. gr., low UNa, low BUN	Restrict water
Dehydration	High sp. gr., low UNa, high BUN	Give water and Na^+
HypoNa with edema	High sp. gr., low UNa, ± high BUN	Restrict Na^+ (and water)
SIADH	High sp. gr., high UNa, low BUN	Restrict water

Abbreviations: sp. gr., urine specific gravity; UNa, urine Na^+ concentration; BUN, blood urea nitrogen; SIADH, syndrome of inappropriate antidiuretic hormone.

TABLE 43. Medications for Hypotension and Shock

Infusion	Infusion Rate	Infusion	Infusion Rate
INOTROPIC DRUGS		**VASODILATORS**	
Dopamine		Nitroprusside	0.5-5.0 μg/kg/minute infusion
Dopaminergic	2.5-5.0 μg/kg/minute	Phentolamine	0.5-5.0 μg/kg/minute infusion
β-adrenergic	5-10 μg/kg/minute	Captopril	0.5-1.0 mg/kg/day divided every 8 hr enterically
β- and α-adrenergic	10-20 μg/kg/minute		
α-adrenergic	>20 μg/kg/minute	Hydralazine	0.1-0.5 mg/kg/dose every 4-6 hr IV
Dobutamine	2.5-20 μg/kg/minute		
Epinephrine	0.05-1.0 μg/kg/minute	Nitroglycerin	1-5 μg/kg/minute infusion
Norepinephrine	0.05-1.0 μg/kg/minute		
Isoproterenol	0.05-1.0 μg/kg/minute	**MAINTENANCE OF DUCTUS ARTERIOSUS**	
Amrinone	Load: 7.5 mg/kg bolus Maintenance: 5-10 μg/kg/minute	Prostaglandin E_1	0.03-0.1 μg/kg/minute infusion

Drug	Dosage	Drug	Dosage
VOLUME EXPANDERS		**DISSEMINATED INTRAVASCULAR COAGULOPATHY**	
Normal saline Ringer's lactate Hetastarch 5% Albumin Purified protein fraction (Plasmanate)	20 ml/kg IV rapid push, repeat as needed; may use 5-10 ml/kg in cardiogenic shock	Fresh frozen plasma	10-20 ml/kg
		Cryoprecipitate	1 unit per 5 kg body weight to increase fibrinogen levels 75 mg/dl
		Heparin	Bolus: 50-100 units/kg, then Infusion: 10-25 units/kg/hr Use cautiously if active bleeding present
ACIDOSIS BUFFERS			
$NaHCO_3$	1 mEq/kg IV (1 ml/kg of a 8.4% solution) *or* mEq $NaHCO_3$ = 0.3 × weight (kg) × base deficit	**OTHER MEDICATIONS** ***Hypoglycemia***	
		Glucose	0.25 g/kg IV bolus
THAM	mEq THAM = 0.25 × weight (kg) × base deficit	**OTHER MEDICATIONS** ***Hyperglycemia***	
		Regular insulin	0.1 unit/kg IV
MUSCLE PARALYSIS*		***Stress Ulcer Prevention***	
Pancuronium	0.1 mg/kg/dose every 1 hr *or* as needed for movement	Ranitidine	1-2 mg/kg per 24 hr divided every 6-8 hr
Vecuronium	0.1 mg/kg/dose every 20-30 minutes *or* 0.1-0.3 mg/kg/hr infusion	Cimetidine	10-40 mg/kg/24 hr divided every 6-8 hr

*Use only for intubation or after intubation is completed.

Table continued on following page

TABLE 43. Medications for Hypotension and Shock *Continued*

Infusion	Infusion Rate	Infusion	Infusion Rate
SEDATIVES†		**SPECIFIC THERAPY FOR ANAPHYLAXIS**	
Benzodiazopines		Epinephrine	Bolus 5-20 μg/kg IV *or* Infusion 0.05-1.0 μg/kg/minute
Diazepam	0.04-0.2 mg/kg/dose every 2-4 hr		
Lorazepam	0.05-0.1 mg/kg/dose every 4-6 hr	Diphenhydramine	1-2 mg/kg slow IV
Midazolam	0.05-0.2 mg/kg/dose every 1-2 hr *or* 0.1-0.5 mg/kg/hr infusion	Dexamethasone	0.25-0.5 mg/kg IV
		or	
		Methylprednisolone	Load: 1-2 mg/kg Maintenance: 0.5 mg/kg/dose every 6 hr
Narcotics			
Morphine sulfate	0.05-0.1 mg/kg/dose every 1-4 hr		
Fentanyl	1-2 μg/kg/dose *or* as infusion 3 μg/kg/hr		

†Use cautiously in hemodynamically unstable patient, as all these drugs can worsen hypotension.

TABLE 44. Laboratory Monitoring Schedule for Infants Receiving Total Parenteral Nutrition

	Baseline and with Any Changes*	Weekly†	Every 2 Weeks
Glucose	X		
Electrolytes	X		
Calcium	X		
Phosphate	X		
Urea nitrogen (BUN)	X		
Triglycerides	X		
Albumin		X	
Fractionated bilirubin		X	
Hemoglobin		X	
Aspartate aminotransferase (AST)		X	
Alanine aminotransferase (ALT)		X	
Alkaline phosphatase			X
Creatinine			X
Gamma-glutamyl transferase (GGT)			X

*Minimum twice weekly.
†More often if clinically indicated.

TABLE 45. Daily Intravenous Requirements for Infants

Component (Energy)	Premature (80-90 kcal/kg)	Term (80-95 kcal/kg)
Glucose: as tolerated for balance of total kcal	6-9 g/kg/day (4-6 mg/kg/minute)	9-12 g/kg/day (6-8 mg/kg/minute)
Maximum carbohydrate	12-14 g/kg/day (8-10 mg/kg/minute)	14-16 g/kg/day (10-12 mg/kg/minute)
Protein: 10-15% of total kcal	Initial intake: 0.5-1.0 g/kg/day Increase 0.5-1.0 g/kg/day as tolerated	
Maximum protein	2.7 g/kg	2.5-3.0 g/kg
Fat: 33-55% of total kcal	Initial: 0.5 g/kg/day, increase 0.5 g/kg/day as tolerated (Minimum requirement to prevent essential fatty acid deficiency is 0.5 g/kg/day)	Initial: 0.5-1.0 g/kg/day
Maximum fat	2.5-3.0 g/kg/day	3.0-3.5 g/kg/day

TABLE 46. Daily Intravenous Major Mineral Requirements (per Kilogram)

Sodium	2-4 mEq (range: 2-8)
Potassium	1-3 mEq (range: 0-5)
Chloride	2-3 mEq (range: 1-5)
Calcium	
Premature	60-100 mg (3-5 mEq)
Term	40-80 mg (2-4 mEq)
Phosphorus	20-45 mg (0.7-1.4 mmol)
Magnesium	0.5-0.9 mEq (6-10 mg)

TABLE 47. Recommendations for Daily Administration of Vitamins and Trace Elements in Infants (per Kilogram)

Vitamins	2 ml of MVI-Pediatric,‡ up to a maximum of 5 ml/day
Zinc	400 μg for infant <37 weeks' gestation 250 μg for term infant <3 months of age
Copper*	20-60 μg
Manganese*	1-5 μg
Chromium†	0.2 μg
Selenium†	2.0 μg
Molybdenum†	0.25 μg (recommended only in long-term total parenteral nutrition)

*Omit in biliary obstruction.
†Reduce in significantly impaired renal function.
‡Rorer Pharmaceuticals, Fort Washington, Pa.
☐ Data from Shils et al: JAMA 241:2050, 1979; and Grune et al: Am J Clin Nutr 48:1324, 1988.

TABLE 48. Drug Treatment of Inflammatory Bowel Disease

Drug	Dose
6-Mercaptopurine	1-1.5 mg/kg/day once daily
Metronidazole	10-15 mg/kg/day three or four times daily
Sulfasalazine	50-70 mg/kg/day three or four times daily

TABLE 49. Patient Guide: Correct Use of a Metered-Dose Inhaler

GENERAL DIRECTIONS

1. Check that there is medicine in the canister at regular intervals.
   a. Put the canister (not the plastic mouthpiece or cap) into a cup of water.
   b. If it sinks to the bottom, it is full. If it floats upright on the surface, it is half full. If it floats sideways on the surface, it is empty.
2. Administer bronchodilator medicines before anti-inflammatory medicines.
3. Consider the use of drug delivery systems or holding chambers (such as InspirEase, Aerochamber, or Inhal-Aid) or other "spacers" or extenders (such as a rolled sheet of notebook paper) if you are using steroid inhalers or if the patient is a young child or someone who may have difficulty accomplishing the optimum technique for inhalation as described below.

Table continued on following page

TABLE 49. Patient Guide: Correct Use of a Metered-Dose Inhaler *Continued*

SPECIFIC STEPS

1. Shake the canister vigorously.
2. Put the mouthpiece on the canister if not using a spacer. If using an AeroChamber, Inhal-Aid, or similar spacer, insert mouthpiece into appropriate opening on the spacer. If using InspirEase, connect mouthpiece to reservoir bag, untwist bag, and insert canister into plastic stem on mouthpiece.
3. Sit up straight or stand up.
4. Take a *big* breath in, then breathe out slowly to the usual place. Do not force air out of your lungs.
5. If not using a spacer, position inhaler with canister above mouthpiece and hold the inhaler with mouthpiece 1 to 2 inches in front of the mouth with mouth wide open. *Do not* put your lips around the mouthpiece.

   If using a spacer, hold mouthpiece of the spacer in your mouth between your teeth with your lips around it.
6. If not using a spacer, begin breathing in *slowly.* Just after you start to breathe in, press down on the canister firmly to release one dose of medicine and keep breathing in.

   If using a spacer, press down on the canister firmly to release one dose of medicine into the spacer and breathe in *slowly.*
7. Finish taking a slow, deep breath. It should take 5 to 10 seconds. Breathe in as deeply as possible.
8. Hold your breath for at least 5 seconds. Try to hold your breath for 10 seconds.
9. If not using a spacer or if using an AeroChamber-type spacer, breathe out slowly through your nose. If using InspirEase, breathe out into the bag and repeat the inhalation cycle as recommended by the manufacturer.
10. If you are experiencing airflow obstruction, subsequent doses of bronchodilator or anti-inflammatory medicines may be more effective if you wait 15 minutes between doses. It is not necessary to wait between doses of anti-inflammatory medicines.
11. If you see the medicine float out of your nose or mouth, it never made it into your lungs! Repeat the dose (but only one more time).
12. Each night, wash mouthpiece (only) and dry thoroughly.

TABLE 50. Inotropic Drugs

Drug	Dose	Effect	Adverse Effects
Dopamine	2.5-5.0 μg/kg/minute	Dopamine receptors; renal and mesenteric vasodilation	
	5.0-10 μg/kg/minute	β_1 increases heart rate	
	10-20 μg/kg/minute	β_2 and α	Tachycardia; arrhythmias
	>720 μg/kg/minute	α; vasoconstriction	
Dobutamine	2.5-20 μg/kg/minute	Predominantly β_1; increases contractility; mild heart rate; mild β_2 effects; vasodilation	Arrhythmias at higher doses
Epinephrine	0.5-1.0 μg/kg/minute	Predominantly β_1 and β_2; some α, especially at higher coses; higher doses may be needed	Arrhythmias; tachycardia; increases myocardial O_2 consumption
Isoproterenol	0.05-1.0 μg/kg/minute	β_1 and β_2; increases heart rate; is common bronchodilator as well as vasodilator	Arrhythmias; tachycardia; increases myocardial O_2 consumption
Norepinephrine	0.05-1.0 μg/kg/minute	Predominantly α; profound vasoconstriction; increases contractility	Decreases peripheal and renal perfusion
Amrinone	Load: 0.75 mg/kg/dose Maintenance: 5-10 μg/kg/minute Maximum: 15 mg/kg/day	Increases contractility; vasodilator	Thrombocytopenia; nausea

TABLE 51. Features of Insulin

Type of Preparation*	Onset (Hours)	Peak (Hours)	Duration at Peak	Intensity
RAPID-ACTING				
Regular P-B, P, B	½	2-4	6-8	Marked
Semilente P-B	½	2-4	10-12	Marked
INTERMEDIATE-ACTING				
NPH P-B, P, B	2	8-10	18-24	Moderate
Lente P-B, P, B	2	8-12	20-26	Moderate
LONG-ACTING				
Ultralente P-B	6	18-24	36+	Mild

*Preparations available from Eli Lilly and Company.
Abbreviations: P-B, pork beef mixture; P, pork only; B, beef only; NPH, neutral protamine Hagedorn (insulin).

TABLE 52. Systemic Drugs Used in Treatment of Acute Lymphoblastic Leukemia

Drug	Dosage	Route	Principal Side Effects
Prednisone	40-120 mg/m^2 daily × 5	p.o.	Immunosuppression, hypertension, hyperglycemia, obesity, mood changes
Vincristine	1.5-2.0 mg/m^2 q 1-3 weeks (2.0 mg maximum)	IV	Peripheral neuropathy, obstipation, alopecia
Doxorubicin or Daunorubicin	30 mg/m^2 q 3 weeks	IV	Myelosuppression, emesis, alopecia, cardiac damage, mucositis
Asparaginase*	25,000 IU/m^2 weekly	IM	Allergic reactions, pancreatitis, coagulopathy, hepatitis, encephalopathy
Methotrexate	30-40 mg/m^2 weekly	IV/IM	Myelosuppression, hepatitis, mucositis
	1 g/m^2 over 24 hours†	IV	
	4 g/m^2 over 1 hour†	IV	
6-Mercaptopurine	50 mg/m^2 daily	p.o.	Myelosuppression, hepatitis, mucositis
	1 g/m^2 over 4-8 hours	IV	

*Alternative preparations (polyethylene glycocylated [PEG] and *Erwinia*) are available from the National Cancer Institute as a substitute for patients with allergic reactions to native *Escherichia coli*.

†Leucovorin rescue required.

TABLE 53. Treatment of Malabsorptive Disorders

Disorder	Treatment
CARBOHYDRATE INTOLERANCE	
Monosaccharide intolerance	
Congenital glucose-galactose malabsorption	Remove glucose and galactose from diet; substitute fructose
Sorbitol and fructose induced diarrhea	Remove offending carbohydrate from diet or substitute juices with lower sorbitol content
Disaccharide intolerance	
Lactase deficiency	Remove lactose from diet; add commercial lactase to milk; take commercial lactase tablets with meals containing lactose
Sucrase-isomaltase deficiency	Avoid sucrose in diet
Polysaccharide	
Amylase deficiency (congenital or secondary to pancreatic damage)	Avoid starch in diet
FAT MALABSORPTION	
Bile salt insufficiency (e.g., cholestasis, terminal ileal resection or dysfunction; primary bile acid malabsorption)	Low-fat diet; medium-chain triglyceride and fat-soluble vitamins A, D, E, K supplementation
Exocrine pancreatic insufficiency (e.g., cystic fibrosis, Shwachman syndrome, chronic pancreatitis)	Pancreatic enzyme replacement (enteric-coated and/or high lipase preparation) with H_2 blocker therapy; fat-soluble vitamin supplements; protein-calorie supplements
Intestinal lymphangiectasia	Medium-chain triglyceride and fat-soluble vitamin supplementation; low-fat diet

Abetalipoproteinemia	Treatment as for lymphangiectasia; vitamin E supplementation, parenterally or as oral alpha-tocopherol polyethylene glycol succinate-1000
Congenital lipase deficiency	Treatment as for exocrine pancreatic insufficiency
SELECTED COMMON DISORDERS CAUSING MUCOSAL INJURY OR INSUFFICIENT ABSORPTIVE SURFACE	
Celiac disease	Gluten-free diet; lactose-free diet until mucosal healing
Inflammatory bowel disease	Anti-inflammatory/immunosuppressive therapy; elemental enteral or possibly parenteral caloric supplementation
Short-bowel syndrome	Treat bacterial overgrowth with antibiotics; medium-chain triglycerides if extensive ileal resection; enteral or parenteral caloric supplementation
Bacterial overgrowth	Treat with appropriate antibiotics (e.g., trimethoprim-sulfamethoxazole, Neomycin)
Parasitic infestation (e.g., *Giardia*)	Treat with metronidazole or other antiprotozoal drug; lactose-free diet, if symptomatic
SPECIFIC MICRONUTRIENT MALABSORPTION	
Acrodermatitis enteropathica (zinc)	Zinc supplementation
Vitamin B_{12} malabsorption	Vitamin B_{12} supplementation usually parenteral; diagnose and treat any vitamin B_{12}-ingesting tapeworm (e.g., *Diphyllobothrium latum*)

TABLE 54. Anticholinesterase Drugs Used for Diagnosis and Treatment of Myasthenia Gravis

Drug	Route	Availability	Dose in Infants	Dose in Children	Comment
Pyridostigmine (Mestinon)	IV, IM	5 mg/ml in 2-ml ampules	0.05-0.15 mg/kg up to q 3-4 hr	1.0-1.5 mg per dose q 3-4 hr	IV/IM dose is equivalent to 1/30 of p.o. dose
Pyridostigmine (Mestinon)	p.o.	12 mg/ml syrup; 60-mg tablet 180 mg sustained-release tablet	4-10 mg up to q 3-4 hr	30-45 mg q 3-8 hr	Each dose is typically effective for 3-4 hr Sustained-release tablets may be most useful at bedtime in adolescent patients
Neostigmine bromide (Prostigmin)	p.o.	15-mg tablet	1-2 mg up to q 2-4 hr	7.5-15 mg up to q 2-4 hr	IV/IM dose is 1/30 of p.o. dose
Edrophonium (Tensilon)	IV	10 mg/ml in 1-mg ampules	0.15-0.2 mg/kg total	0.2 mg/kg total; maximum, 10 mg	For diagnosis only. Give 1/5 total dose as test dose; if tolerated, give remainder incrementally. Monitor BP and heart rate. Atropine (0.01 mg/kg up to 0.4 mg) can block or reverse muscarinic effects.

Abbreviations: IV, intravenously; IM, intramuscularly; q, every; p.o., by mouth; BP, blood pressure.

TABLE 55. Treatment of Neonatal Withdrawal Syndrome

Drug	Dosage
Paregoric	3-6 drops every 4 to 6 hours, p.o.
Laudanum (0.4%)	3-6 drops every 4 to 6 hours, p.o.
Chlorpromazine	2-3 mg/kg/day every 6 hours, p.o.
Phenobarbital	3-6 mg/kg/day every 6 hours, p.o.

TABLE 56. Drugs Useful for Control of Nausea and Vomiting

Drug	How Supplied	Principal Side Effects
ANTIHISTAMINES		
Promethazine (Phenergan) Child: 1 mg/kg/dose q 4-6 hr p.o. or IM Adult: 25 mg p.o. or IM	Syrup: 6.25 mg/5 ml or 25 mg/5 ml Tablets: 12.5, 25, 50 mg Suppository: 12.5, 25, 50 mg Injection: 25 mg/1 ml	Headache Abdominal pain Urinary urgency Blood pressure changes Extrapyramidal and anticholinergic side effects
Dimenhydrinate (Dramamine) Child: 1.25 mg/kg/dose p.o. or IM, q.i.d. Adult: 50-100 mg/dose p.o. or IM q.i.d., 100 mg p.r. q.i.d.	Injection: 50 mg/ml Liquid: 12.5 mg/4 ml Tablets: 50 mg Suppository: 100 mg	Drowsiness Atropine-like effects
DOPAMINE ANTAGONISTS		
Metoclopramide (Reglan) Child: 0.1 mg/kg/dose p.o., IM, or IV q 6 hr Adult: 10 mg p.o. IM or IV q 6 hr	Injection: 5 mg/ml Syrup: 5 mg/ml Tablets: 10 mg	Extrapyramidal restlessness, sedation, lowered threshold to seizure
Thiethylperazine (Torecan) Child: 5 mg p.o. q.i.d. if <50 kg, 10 mg if >50 kg Adult: 10-30 mg p.o. q.i.d. 10 mg IM t.i.d.	Injection: 10 mg/2 ml Tablet: 10 mg Suppository: 10 mg	Extrapyramidal and anticholinergic effects

Perphenazine (Trilafon) Adult: 8-16 mg p.o. b.i.d.-q.i.d. 8-10 mg IV or IM q 6 hr or as continuous infusion	Tablets: 2, 4, 8, 16 mg Injection: 5 mg/ml	Extrapyramidal and anticholinergic effects
Prochlorperazine (Compazine) Child (>10 kg) 0.05 mg/kg IM q 6 hr or 0.1 mg/kg p.r. or p.o. q 6 hr Adult 5-10 mg/dose IM or p.o. 6 hr or 25 mg p.r. b.i.d.	Injection: 5 mg/ml Syrup: 5 mg/5 ml Oral concentrate: 10 mg/ml Suppository: 2.5, 5, 25 mg	Extrapyramidal more common than anticholinergic, sedation, dysphoria, orthostatic hypotension, lowered seizure threshold
MISCELLANEOUS		
Phosphorated carbohydrate solution (Emetrol) Child: 1-2 tsp. q 15 minutes until nausea subsides Adult: 1-2 Tbsp. q 15 minutes until nausea subsides	Liquid: 1.87 g dextrose 1.87 g fructose 21.5 mg phosphoric acid/5 ml	Nontoxic
Lorazepam (Ativan) Usual dose 2-3 mg/day in divided doses	Tablets: 0.5, 1, 2 mg	For psychogenic vomiting
Diazepam (Valium) Child: 1-2½ mg, 3 or 4 times daily Adult: 2-10 mg, 3 or 4 times daily	Tablets: 2, 5, 10 mg	For psychogenic vomiting

Abbreviations: p.o., by mouth; IM, intramuscular; IV, intravenous; q, every; b.i.d., twice a day; q.i.d., four times a day; t.i.d., three times a day; p.r., per rectum.

TABLE 57. Assessment of the Clinical Severity of Neonatal Withdrawal

	Mild	Moderate	Severe
Vomiting	Spitting up	Extensive vomiting for 3 successive feedings	Vomiting associated with imbalance of serum electrolytes
Diarrhea	Watery stools <4 times/day	Watery stools 5-6 times/day for 3 days; no electrolyte imbalance	Diarrhea associated with imbalance of serum electrolytes
Weight loss	<10% of birth weight	10-15% of birth weight	>15% of birth weight
Irritability	Minimal	Marked but relieved by cuddling or feeding	Unrelieved by cuddling or feeding
Tremors or twitching	Mild tremors when stimulated	Marked tremors or twitching when stimulated	Convulsions
Tachypnea	60-80/minute	80-100/minute	>100 breaths/minute and associated with respiratory alkalosis

TABLE 58. Medications for Neonatal Resuscitation

Medication	Concentrations to Administer	Preparation	Dosage and Route	Total Dose per Infant			Rate and Precautions
				Weight (kg)	Total Dose	Total (ml)	
Epinephrine	1:10,000	1 ml	0.1-0.3 ml/kg IV or ET	1		0.1-0.3	Give rapidly. Make dilute with normal saline to 1-2 ml if giving ET.
				2		0.2-0.6	
				3		0.3-0.9	
				4		0.4-1.2	
Volume expanders	Whole blood	40 ml	10 ml/kg IV	1		10	Give over 5-10 minutes
	5% Albumin			2		20	
	Normal saline			3		30	
	Ringer's lactate			4		40	
Sodium bicarbonate	0.5 mEq/ml (4.2% solution)	20 ml *or* two 10-ml prefilled syringes	2 mEq/kg IV	1	2 mEq	4	Give *slowly*, over at least 2 minutes
				2	4 mEq	8	
				3	6 mEq	12	Give only if infant being effectively ventilated
				4	8 mEq	16	
Naloxone	0.4 mg/ml	1 ml	0.1 mg/kg (0.25 ml/kg) IV, ET, IM, SQ	1	0.1 mg	0.25	Give rapidly
				2	0.2 mg	0.50	IV, ET preferred
				3	0.3 mg	0.75	IM, SQ acceptable
				4	0.4 mg	1.00	

Table continued on following page

TABLE 58. Medications for Neonatal Resuscitation *Continued*

Medication	Concentrations to Administer	Preparation	Dosage and Route	Total Dose per Infant: Weight (kg)	Total Dose	Total (ml)	Rate and Precautions
	1.0 mg/ml	1 ml	0.1 mg/kg (0.1 ml/kg) IV, ET, IM, SQ	1	0.1 mg	0.1	
				2	0.2 mg	0.2	
				3	0.3 mg	0.3	
				4	0.4 mg	0.4	
					Total (μg/min)		
Dopamine	$\frac{6 \times \text{weight (kg)} \times \text{desired dose } (\mu g/kg/minute)}{\text{desired fluid (ml/hr)}} =$	mg of dopamine per 100 ml of solution	Begin at 5 μg/kg minute (may increase to 20 μg/kg/minute if necessary) IV	1	5-20		Give as a continuous infusion using an infusion pump
				2	10-40		Monitor HR and BP closely
				3	15-60		Seek consultation
				4	20-80		

Abbreviations: IV, intravenous; ET, endotracheal; IM, intramuscular; SQ, subcutaneous; HR, heart rate; BP, blood pressure.

TABLE 59. Local Anesthetics for Ocular Use

Generic Name	Trade Name	Concentration
Tetracaine solution	Pontocaine	0.5%
Tetracaine ointment	Pontocaine	0.5%
Proparacaine solution	AK-Taine	0.5%
	Alcaine	0.5%
	I-Paracaine	0.5%
	Kainair	0.5%
	Ophthaine	0.5%
	Ophthetic	0.5%

TABLE 60. Topical Antibiotic and Sulfonamide Eye Preparations

Generic Name	Trade Name	Concentration
DROPS		
Chloramphenicol solution	Chloromycetin	0.16–0.5%
	AK-Chlor	0.5%
	Chloroptic	0.5%
	Ophthochlor	0.5%
Ciprofloxacin	Ciloxan	0.35%
Gentamicin solution	Garamycin	0.3%
	Genoptic	0.3%
	Gentacidin	0.3%
	Gentrasul	0.3%
	Gent-AK	0.3%
Norfloxacin	Chibroxin	0.3%
Polymixin-B solution		10,000–25,000 U/ml
Sulfacetamide solution	AK-Sulf	10% & 15%
	AK-Sulf Forte	30%
	Bleph-10	10%
	Isopto Cetamide	15%
	Ophthacet	10%
	Sodium Sulamyd	10% & 30%
	Sulf-10	10%
	Sulfair-15	15%
	Sulten-10	10%
Sulfisoxazole solution	Gantrisin	4%
Tetracycline suspension	Achromycin	1%
Tobramycin solution	Tobrex	0.3%
OINTMENTS		
Bacitracin	AK-Tracin	500 U/g
Chloramphenicol	AK-Chlor	10 mg/g
	Chloromycetin	10 mg/g
	Chloroptic S.O.P.	10 mg/g
Chlortetracycline	Aureomycin	10 mg/g
Erythromycin	AK-Mycin	5 mg/g
	Ilotycin	5 mg/g
Gentamicin	Garamycin	3 mg/g
	Genoptic S.O.P.	3 mg/g
	Gentacidin	3 mg/g
	Gentrasul	3 mg/g
	Gent-AK	3 mg/g

Table continued on following page

TABLE 60. Topical Antibiotic and Sulfonamide Eye Preparations
Continued

Generic Name	Trade Name	Concentration
Sulfacetamide	AK-Sulf	10%
	Bleph-10 S.O.P.	10%
	Cetamide	10%
	Sodium Sulamyd	10%
Sulfisoxazole	Gantrisin	4%
Tetracycline	Achromycin	10 mg/g
Tobramycin	Tobrex	3 mg/g

TABLE 61. Topical Antimicrobial Combination Eye Preparations

Generic Name	Trade Name
DROP	
Polymyxin B + neomycin	Statrol
Polymyxin B + neomycin + gramicidin	AK-Spore
	Neocidin
	Neosporin
	Neotricin
Polymyxin B + trimethoprim	Polytrim
Polymyxin B + trimethoprim	Polytrim
OINTMENTS	
Polymyxin B + bacitracin	AK-Poly-Bac
	Polysporin
Polymyxin B + neomycin	Statrol
Polymyxin B + bacitracin + neomycin	AK-Spore
	Neosporin
	Neotal
	Mycitracin
Polymyxin B + chloramphenicol	Chloromyxin
Polymyxin B + oxytetracycline	Terramycin

TABLE 62. Topical Antimicrobial-Corticosteroid Eye Preparations

Generic Name	Trade Name
DROPS	
Chloramphenicol + hydrocortisone (suspension)	Chloromycetin-hydrocortisone
Gentamicin + prednisolone (suspension)	Pred-G
Neomycin + hydrocortisone (suspension)	AK-Neo-Cort Cor-Oticin Neo-Cortef Ortho Drops
Neomycin + dexamethasone (solution)	Neo-Decadron
Neomycin + polymyxin B + hydrocortisone (suspension)	Cortisporin Triple-Gen
Neomycin + polymyxin B + prednisolone (suspension)	Poly-Pred
Neomycin + polymyxin B + dexamethasone (suspension)	AK-Trol Dexacidin Infectrol Maxitrol
Sulfacetamide + fluorometholone (suspension)	FML-S
Sulfacetamide + prednisolone (suspension)	AK-Cide Blephamide Isopto Cetapred Metimyd Ophtha P/S Or-Toptic M Predamide Predsulfair Sulfamide Sulphrin
Sulfacetamide + prednisolone (solution)	Optimyd Vasocidin
Tobramycin + dexamethasone (suspension)	TobraDex
OINTMENTS	
Chloramphenicol + polymyxin B + hydrocortisone	Ophthocort
Neomycin + dexamethasone	Neo-Decadron
Neomycin + polymyxin B + bacitracin + hydrocortisone	Coracin Cortisporin

Table continued on following page

TABLE 62. Topical Antimicrobial-Corticosteroid Eye Preparations *Continued*

Generic Name	Trade Name
Sulfacetamide + prednisolone	AK-Cide Blephamide S.O.P. Cetapred Metimyd Predsulfair Vasocidin

TABLE 63. Topical Corticosteroid Eye Preparations

Generic Name	Trade Name	Concentration
DROPS		
Dexamethasone alcohol (suspension)	Maxidex	0.1%
Dexamethasone sodium phosphate (solution)	AK-Dex	0.1%
	Baldex	0.1%
	Decadron	0.1%
Fluorometholone (suspension)	FML	0.1%
	Fluor-Op	0.1%
	FML Forte	0.25%
Medrysone (suspension)	HMS	1%
Prednisolone acetate (suspension)	Econopred	0.125%
	Econopred Plus	1%
	Pred Mild	0.12%
	Pred Forte	1%
Prednisolone sodium phosphate (solution)	AK-Pred	0.125% & 1%
	Inflamase Mild	0.125%
	Inflamase Forte	1%
	Metreton	0.5%
OINTMENTS		
Dexamethasone sodium phosphate	AK-Dex	0.05%
	Baldex	0.05%
	Decadron	0.05%
	Maxidex	0.05%
Fluorometholone	FML	0.1%

TABLE 64. Topical Vasoconstrictor, Astringent, and Antihistaminic Preparations

Generic Name	Trade Name
VASOCONSTRICTORS	
Naphazoline (0.1%)	AK-Con
	Albalon
	Muro's Opcon
	Nafazair
	Naphcon Forte
	Opcon
	Vasocon Regular
Naphazoline (0.03%)	Comfort Eye Drops
Naphazoline (0.025%)	Naphazoline
Naphazoline (0.02%)	VasoClear
Naphazoline (0.012%)	Allerest
	Clear Eyes
	Degest 2
	Estivin II
	Naphcon
Phenylephrine (0.12%)	AK-Nefrin
	Isopto Frin
	Prefrin
Tetrahydrozoline (0.05%)	Murine Plus
	Optigene
	Soothe
	Visine
VASOCONSTRICTORS WITH ASTRINGENT OR ANTIHISTAMINE	
Naphazoline (0.02%) + zinc sulfate (0.25%)	VasoClear A
Naphazoline (0.05%) + antazoline (0.5%)	Albalon-A
	Vasocon-A
Naphazoline (0.025%) + pheniramine (0.3%)	AK-Con-A
	Opcon-A
	Naphcon-A
Phenylephrine (0.125%) + pheniramine maleate (0.5%)	AK-Vernacon
Phenylephrine (0.12%) + pyrilamine (0.1%)	Prefrin-A
Phenylephrine (0.12%) + zinc sulfate (0.25%)	Phenylzin
	Zincfrin
Tetrahydrozoline (0.05%) + zinc sulfate (0.25%)	Visine A.C.

TABLE 65. Recommended Antibiotic Regimens for Treatment of Pelvic Inflammatory Disease

- Cefoxitin (2.0 g IV every 6 hr) *or* Cefotetan (2.0 g IV every 12 hr)

  plus

  Doxycycline (100 mg IV or p.o. every 12 hr)

Continue treatment for a total of 4 days *and* until the patient is afebrile for at least 48 hr. The patient is then discharged on doxycycline (100 mg p.o. b.i.d.) to complete 10–14 days of therapy.

This regimen provides optimal coverage of both *Neisseria gonorrhoeae,* including penicillinase-producing *N. gonorrhoeae,* and *Chlamydia trachomatis.* It may not provide optimum anaerobic coverage for patients with tubo-ovarian abscess or IUD-associated PID.

or

- Clindamycin (900 mg IV every 8 hr)

  plus

  Gentamicin (2.0 mg/kg loading dose IV, then 1.5 mg/kg IV every 8 hr)

Continue treatment for a total of 4 days *and* until the patient is afebrile for at least 48 hr. The patient is then discharged on either clindamycin (450 mg p.o. q.i.d.) or doxycycline (100 mg p.o. b.i.d.) to complete 10–14 days of therapy.

This regimen provides excellent coverage of anaerobes and gram-negative organisms. Although it may theoretically be suboptimal for treatment of *C. trachomatis* and *N. gonorrhoeae,* a recent study has shown this regimen to be equivalent to the cefoxitin-doxycycline regimen in eradicating *N. gonorrhoeae* and *C. trachomatis.*

Abbreviations: p.o., by mouth; b.i.d., twice a day; IUD, intrauterine device; PID, pelvic inflammatory disease; q.i.d., four times a day.

TABLE 66. Antibiotic Dosing Guidelines for the Treatment of Peritonitis in Pediatric Patients Receiving Continuous Peritoneal Dialysis*

	Half-Life			Dose‡		
				Initial		Maintenance
	Normal	ESRD	CAPD	mg/kg	mg/L of Dialysate	mg/L of Dialysate
AMINOGLYCOSIDES						
Amikacin†	1.6	39	ND	5.0–7.5 IV/IP	—	6–7.5
Gentamicin†	2.2	53	32	1.5–1.7 IV/IP	—	4–6
Netilmicin†	2.1	42	ND	1.5–2.0 IV/IP	—	4–6
Tobramycin†	2.5	58	36	1.5–1.7 IV/IP	—	4–6
CEPHALOSPORINS						
Cefamandole	1.0	10	8.0	—	500	ND
Cefazolin	2.2	28	27	—	250–500	125–250
Cefoperazone	1.8	2.3	2.2	—	1000	500
Cefotaxime	0.9	2.5	2.4		1000	250
Cefoxitin	0.8	20	15	—	500	100
Ceftazidime	1.8	26	16	—	500	125
Ceftizoxime	1.6	28	11	—	500	125

Ceftriaxone	8.0	15	13	—	500	ND
Cefuroxime	1.3	18	15	—	750	250
Cephalothin	0.2	3.7	ND	—	1000	250
Moxalactam	2.2	20	16	—	500	ND
Cephradine	0.9	12	ND	—	250	125–250
Cephalexin	0.8	19	9	12.5 p.o.	—	12.5 mg/kg per dose q 8 hr p.o.
PENICILLINS						
Ampicillin	1.2	15	ND	—	250	50
Azlocillin	0.9	5.1	ND	—	250	250
Ticarcillin	1.2	15	ND	75 IV	—	75 mg/kg per dose q 12 hr IV
VANCOMYCIN AND OTHERS						
Vancomycin†	6.9	161	83	15 IV/IP	—	25–30
Clindamycin	2.8	2.8	ND	—	150	150

*Continuous peritoneal dialysis—CAPD or CCPD.

†Blood levels should be obtained periodically to avoid toxicity.

‡Current recommendations are adapted from the adult literature and are subject to change as/if new information on pediatric dosage becomes available.

Abbreviations: ESRD, end-stage renal disase; CAPD, continuous ambulatory peritoneal dialysis; IV/IP, intravenously/intraperitoneally; q, every; p.o., by mouth; ND, no data.

TABLE 67. Empiric Intraperitoneal Antibiotic Dosages for Suspected CAPD or CCPD Peritonitis

	Loading Dose	Maintenance Dose
Cephalothin* *plus*	25 mg/kg (in a single exchange)	250 mg/L
Tobramycin*	1.7 mg/kg (in a single exchange)	4 to 6 mg/L

*May be mixed in dialysis fluid without affecting potency.
Abbreviations: CAPD, continuous ambulatory peritoneal dialysis; CCPD, continuous cycling peritoneal dialysis.

TABLE 68. Antihistamines for Treatment of Physical Allergy

Antihistamine Class (Histamine Receptor)	Drug (Trade Name)	Usual Dose, 27-kg Child (Dose by Weight)
Ethanolamine	Diphenhydramine (Benadryl) (more sedative)	12.5–50 mg 3 × daily (5 mg/kg/24 hr—not to exceed 300 mg/24 hr)
Ataractic (H_1)	Hydroxyzine (Atarax, Vistaril) (more sedative)	10–25 mg 3 × daily for children < 6 yr; 50 mg maximum total daily dose
Piperidine-butanol (H_1) (second generation)	Terfenadine* (Seldane) (no sedative) (less sedative)	60 mg 2 × daily for children ≥ 12 yr; not recommended for children < 12 yr but commonly used
Benzimidazole amine (H_1) (second generation)	Astemizole* (Hismanal) (not sedating)	10 mg q A.M. (1 × daily); not recommended for children < 12 yr
Alkylamine (H_1)	1. Chlorpheniramine (Chlor-Trimeton, Teldrin) 2. Brompheniramine (Dimetane) (less sedative)	2–8 mg 3 × daily
Benzhydryl ether (H_1)	Clemastine fumarate (Tavist) (less sedative)	1.34-mg tablet 2 × daily; not recommended for children < 12 yr of age 0.5 mg/5 ml (syrup) 2–3 × daily—safety confirmed in children 6–12 yr

Table continued on following page

TABLE 68. Antihistamines for Treatment of Physical Allergy
Continued

Antihistamine Class (Histamine Receptor)	Drug (Trade Name)	Usual Dose, 27-kg Child (Dose by Weight)
Piperidine (H_1)	1. Cyproheptadine (Periactin) 2. Azatadine (Optimine)	2–4 mg 3–4 × daily (0.25 mg/kg/24 hr) 1–2 mg 2 × daily; not recommended for children < 12 yr
Phenothiazine (H_1)	Promethazine (Phenergan)	6.15–12.5 mg 3 × daily
Ethylenediamine (H_1)	Tripelennamine (PBZ)	25–50 mg 3 × daily (5 mg/kg/24 hr—not to exceed 300 mg/24 hr)
Thioguanidine (H_2)	Cimetidine (Tagamet)	20–40 mg/kg/24 hr; very limited experience in children < 16 yr
Ethenediamine (H_2)	Ranitidine (Zantac)	Dosage not established in children; see manufacturer's recommendations
Ataractics (H_1, H_2)	Doxepin (Sinequan)	10–25 mg 2 × daily for children ≥ 12 yr as a single drug; not to exceed 75 mg/24 hr; not recommended for children < 12 yr

*Warning: Concomitant use with erythromycin or ketoconazole may raise blood levels and increase risk of cardiac arrhythmias.

TABLE 69. Medications Used in Childhood Psychiatric Disorders

Drug	Indication
Antidepressants	
Fluoxetine (Prozac)	Obsessive-compulsive disorder
Clomipramine	Obsessive-compulsive disorder
Amitriptyline	Depression; Attention deficit hyperactivity disorder
Imipramine	Separation anxiety disorder; Depression; Attention deficit hyperactivity disorder
Desipramine	Separation anxiety disorder; Depression; Attention deficit hyperactivity disorder
Benzodiazepines	Overanxious disorder; Avoidant disorder; Panic disorder; Anticipatory anxiety disorder
Antihistamines	
Diphenhydramine	Anxiety disorder
Hydroxyzine	Anxiety disorder
Buspirone (BuSpar)	Overanxious disorder
Beta-blockers	Extreme agitation and aggression
Monoamine oxidase inhibitors	Depression
Lithium carbonate	Bipolar disorder; Depression; Conduct disorder with irritability and mood lability
Stimulants	
Methylphenidate (Ritalin)	Attention deficit hyperactivity disorder
Dextroamphetamine (Dexedrine)	Attention deficit hyperactivity disorder
Pemoline (Cylert)	Attention deficit hyperactivity disorder
Clonidine	Attention deficit hyperactivity disorder

TABLE 70. Recommended Dietary Allowances (RDA)* for Caloric Intake of Infants, Children, and Adolescents

Category	Age (Years)	REE† (kcal/day)	Caloric Allowance		
			kcal/kg/day‡	kcal/day	Range
Infants	0.0–0.5	320	108	kg × 108	(520–780)
	0.5–1.0	500	98	kg × 98	(680–1020)
Children	1–3	740	102	1300	(1040–1560)
	4–6	950	90	1800	(1440–2160)
	7–10	1130	70	2000	(1600–2400)
Males	11–14	1440	55	2500	(2000–3000)
	15–18	1760	45	3000	(2400–3600)
Females	11–14	1310	47	2200	(1760–2640)
	15–18	1370	40	2200	(1760–2640)

*The RDAs for protein, vitamins, and minerals appear in the section "Vitamin deficiencies and excesses."

†Resting energy expenditure (REE) is similar to basal metabolic rate.

‡The calculation of kcal/kg/day in children ≥ 3 years of age is based on the average of a wide range of acceptable intakes. Appropriate rates of growth may occur at energy intake levels above and below this estimate.

TABLE 71. Choice of Drug and Seizure Type

Drug	Seizure Type	Dose (mg/kg per 24 Hours)	Preparation	Frequency per 24 Hours	Plasma Level (μg/ml)	Half-Life (Hours)
Carbamazepine (Tegretol)	Partial Secondarily generalized	10–25	200 mg tablets 100 mg chewable tablets 100 mg/5 ml suspension	2 or 3	4–12	6–12
Ethosuximide (Zarontin)	Absence	15–40	250 mg capsules 250 mg/ml liquid	2 to 3	40–100	24–36
Phenobarbital	Primary generalized Secondary generalized Partial Status	4–8	Tablets 15 mg, 30 mg, 60 mg; 20 mg/5 ml suspension	1 or 2	15–40	48–100
Phenytoin (Dilantin)	Primary generalized Secondary generalized Partial	4–8	100 mg capsules 50 mg chewable tablets	1 or 2	10–20	6–30

	Status		100 mg/5 ml suspension			
Primidone (Mysoline)	Primary generalized Secondary generalized	10–25	50 mg tablets 250 mg tablets 250 mg/5 ml suspension	3–4	5–12	10–36
Valproate (Depakene)	Primary generalized Absence Myoclonic Partial Atypical absence	20–60	250 mg capsules 125, 250, 500 mg tablets 125 mg sprinkle capsules 250 mg/5 ml liquid	2–3	40–150	6–12
Clonazepam (Klonopin)	Absence Primary generalized Partial Myoclonic	0.05–0.3	0.5, 1 and 2 mg tablets	2–3		24–36

TABLE 72. Treatment for Skin Infections in the Neonate

Drug	Indication	Route	Dose
Acyclovir	Neonatal herpes	IV	30 mg/kg/24 hr in 3 divided doses × 10–14 days
Penicillin			
Aqueous	Congenital syphilis	IM or IV	50,000 units/kg/24 hr in 2 divided doses × 10 days
Procaine	Congenital syphilis	IM	50,000 units/kg/24 hr daily × 10 days
Ampicillin	Neonatal listerial infection	IM or IV	50–75 mg/kg/24 hr in 2–3 divided doses
Methicillin	Neonatal staphylococcal infection	IM or IV	50–100 mg/kg/24 hr in 2–3 divided doses
Vancomycin	Neonatal staphylococcal infection	p.o. or IV	30–45 mg/kg/24 hr in 2 or 3 divided doses
Prednisone	Cavernous hemangioma	p.o.	2–3 mg/kg per 24 hr once daily × 4 weeks

TABLE 73. Treatment of Status Epilepticus

Drug	Dose	May Be Repeated?
FIRST RESORT		
Diazepam	0.2–0.4 mg/kg IV at 1 mg/minute, maximum dose 10 mg	Yes, after 15 minutes
Lorazepam	0.5–0.1 mg/kg IV over 1–2 minutes, maximum dose 5 mg	Yes, but loses effectiveness
Phenobarbital	20 mg/kg IV given at 100 mg/minute, maximum dose 300 mg	Yes
Phenytoin	20 mg/kg IV at 50 mg/minute, maximum dose 1000 mg	No
LAST RESORT		
Pentobarbital	20 mg/kg loading dose, then continuous IV drip of 1–2 mg/kg/hour	

TABLE 74. Intravenous Therapy for Complicated Urinary Tract Infections

Indication	Antibiotic	Dose
Neonates* and young infants	Ampicillin	75–100 mg/kg/day IV in 4 divided doses
	plus	
	Gentamicin†	7.5 mg/kg/day IV in 3 divided doses × 10–14 days
Complicated UTI‡ (pyelonephritis) in older infants and children	Ampicillin	100–200 mg/kg/day IV in 4 divided doses
	plus	
	Gentamicin†	6–7.5 mg/kg/day IV in 3 doses
	or	
	Cefotaxime	100–200 mg/kg/day IV in 3 divided doses
	or	
	Ceftriaxone	50–75 mg/kg/day IV or IM in a single or 2 divided doses

*Doses must be adjusted for neonates younger than 1 week old.
†Optimal management requires monitoring of serum concentrations.
‡See text for antibiotic therapy for *Pseudomonas* and multiply resistant organisms.

TABLE 75. Oral Antimicrobial Therapy for Urinary Tract Infections (UTIs) in Children

Indication	Antibiotic	Dose
Asymptomatic bacteriuria or uncomplicated UTI (cystitis)	Amoxicillin	40–50 mg/kg/day p.o. in 3 divided doses
	or	
	Sulfisoxazole	120–150 mg/kg/day p.o. in 4 divided doses
	or	
	TMP/SMX	TMP 10 mg/kg/day + SMX 50 mg/kg/day p.o. in 2 divided doses
	or	
	Cephalexin	50 mg/kg/day p.o. in 4 divided doses
	or	
	Cefixime	3 mg/kg/day p.o. given once daily
Chemoprophylaxis	TMP/SMX	TMP 2 mg/kg/day + SMX 10 mg/kg/day p.o. every 1–2 days at bedtime
	or	
	Nitrofurantoin	1–2 mg/kg/day p.o. every day at bedtime

TABLE 76. Management of Dysfunctional Uterine Bleeding

MILD DUB: inconvenient, unpredictable bleeding/Hb > 12 g/dl
- Reassurance
- Fe supplementation
- Consider oral contraceptive
- Reevaluate every 3–6 months

MODERATE DUB: irregular, prolonged, heavy bleeding/Hb > 10 g/dl
- Hormonal therapy:
  - Provera (10 mg daily for 5–7 days every 35–40 days)
    or
  - Oral contraceptives
- Fe supplementation
- Menstrual calendar
- Reevaluate in 1–2 months

SEVERE DUB: irregular, heavy prolonged bleeding/Hb < 10 g/dl
- Not actively bleeding
  - Oral contraceptive
  - Fe supplementation
  - Reevaluate in 1–3 months
- Active mild to moderate bleeding
  - Ovral, 1 tablet every 6 hr for 24–48 hr, tapered over the following week to 1 tablet daily
  - Fe supplementation
  - Reevaluate in 1 week, then in 1–3 months
- Active heavy bleeding
  - Hospitalize
  - Transfuse if necessary
  - Hormonal therapy:
    - Ovral, 1 tablet every 6 hr for 24–48 hr, tapered over the week to 1 tablet daily *or* Premarin (20–25 mg IV every 4 hr) for maximum 6 doses with concurrent Ovral (1 tablet every 6 hr, tapered over the following week to 1 tablet daily)
      followed by
    - Oral contraceptive for 6 to 12 months (consider continuous regimen, i.e., without placebos, until Hb normalizes)
    - D & C if hormonal therapy fails
    - Re-evaluate 1–2 weeks and 1 month after discharge, then in 1–3 months until menstrual pattern and Hb stable

Abbreviations: DUB, dysfunctional uterine bleeding; Hb, hemoglobin; Fe, iron; D & C, dilatation and curettage.

☐ Adapted from Muram D. Vaginal bleeding in childhood and adolescence. *In* Menstrual Cycle Disorders, Obstet Gynecol Clin North Am 17:405, 1990.

TABLE 77. Formulation of Vasoactive Infusions

Drug	Action	Mixture Formula
Dopamine	Inotrope	6 × weight (kg) = mg in 100 ml of D_5W
Dobutamine	Inotrope	
Nitroprusside	Vasodilator	
Phentolamine	Vasodilator	1 ml/hr = 1 μg/kg/minute
Epinephrine	Inotrope	0.6 × weight (kg) = mg in 100 ml of D_5W
Norepinephrine	Inotrope	
Prostaglandin E_1	Ductus arteriosus dilator	1 ml/hr = 0.1 μg/kg/minute

Abbreviation: D_5W, 5 per cent dextrose in water.

TABLE 78. Considerations for Vitamin and Mineral Supplementation for Healthy Children

	Vitamins				Minerals		
	D	C	B_{12}	Folate	Iron	Calcium	Fluoride*
INFANTS (BIRTH TO 6 MONTHS)							
Breast milk	+	–	–	–	–	–	±
Vegetarian breast milk	+	–	+	–	–	–	±
Commercial formula	–	–	–	–	–	–	±
Evaporated milk†	–	+	–	–	–	–	±
Goat's milk	+	+	–	+	+	–	±
Cow's milk†‡	–	+	–	–	+	–	±
OLDER INFANTS (6 TO 12 MONTHS)	–	–	–	–	+§	–	±
CHILDREN							
Healthy	–	–	–	–	–	–	±
Lactose-intolerant	–	–	–	–	–	+‖	±
Vegetarian¶	±	–	±	–	+	±	±

ADOLESCENTS#							
Healthy	–	–	–	–	±	±	±
Lactose-intolerant	–	–	–	–	±	+‖	±
Vegetarian¶	±	–	±	–	+	±	±
Pregnant	–	–	–	+	+	+	±

*Depending on fluoride content of local water supply.

†Assuming vitamin D-fortified evaporated milk and whole cow's milk.

‡Inadequate in linolenic acid: may cause gastrointestinal blood loss.

§Usually supplied by infant cereal or iron-fortified commercial formula.

‖Calcium-containing dairy products are often omitted or limited with lactose intolerance.

¶Supplementation requirements depend on type of vegetarian diet (e.g., use of eggs, milk products) consumed.

#Adolescent diets are frequently inadequate in calcium and iron.

Key: +, supplementation needed; ±, supplementation may be needed; –, not needed.

REFERENCES FOR TABLE 15, PP. 140 AND 141

(1) Addiego JE, Jr., Gomperts E, Liu S-L, et al: Treatment of hemophilia A with a highly purified factor VIII concentrate prepared by anti-FVIIIs immunoaffinity chromatography. *Thrombos Haemostas* 67:19–27, 1992.

(2) Horowitz MS, Horowitz B, Rooks C, Hilgartner MW: Virus safety of solvent/detergent-treated antihaemophilic factor concentrate. *Lancet* 2:186–188, 1988.

(3) Schimpf K, Mannucci PM, Kreutz W, et al: Absence of hepatitis after treatment with a pasteurized factor VIII concentrate in patients with hemophilia and no previous transfusions. *N Engl J Med,* 316:918–922, 1987.

(4) Bergman, G (personal communication; manuscript in preparation—as of 5-20-93, 26 previously untreated patients followed at least 6 months and 19 at least 12 months with no instance of viral illness or seroconversions to HCV, HAV, HIV, CMV, EBV, HBV).

(5) Study Group of the UK Haemophilia Center Directors on Surveillance of Virus Transmission by Concentrates. Effect of dry heating of coagulation factor concentrates at 80° C for 72 hrs on transmission of non-A, non-B hepatitis. *Lancet* 2:184–816, 1988.

(6) Kernoff PBA, Miller EJ, Savidge GF, et al: Reduced risk of non-A, non-B hepatitis after a first exposure to 'wet-heated' factor FVIII concentrate. *Br J Haemotol,* 67:207–211, 1987.

(7) Waytes, T (personal communication; manuscript in preparations—data have been published in abstract form).

(8) Mannucci PM, Zanetti AR, Colombo M and the Study Group of the Foundazione dell' Emophilia: Prospective study of hepatitis after factor VIII concentrate exposed to hot vapour. *Br J Haematol,* 68:427–430, 1988.

(9) Kasper CK, Lusher JM, and Transfusion Practices Committee, AABB: Recent Evolution of Clotting Factor Concentrates for Hemophilia A and B. *Transfusion* 33:422–434, 1993.

Index

Note: Page numbers followed by t refer to tables.

Note: Page numbers followed by t refer to tables.

Note: Page numbers followed by t refer to tables.

Note: Page numbers followed by t refer to tables.

D

Note: Page numbers followed by t refer to tables.

E

Note: Page numbers followed by t refer to tables.

Note: Page numbers followed by t refer to tables.

Note: Page numbers followed by t refer to tables.

I

J

K

Note: Page numbers followed by t refer to tables.

L

M

Note: Page numbers followed by t refer to tables.

Note: Page numbers followed by t refer to tables.

O

Note: Page numbers followed by t refer to tables.

Note: Page numbers followed by t refer to tables.

Note: Page numbers followed by t refer to tables.

Note: Page numbers followed by t refer to tables.

Note: Page numbers followed by t refer to tables.

Note: Page numbers followed by t refer to tables.

Note: Page numbers followed by t refer to tables.